CBT FOR DEPRESSION
IN CHILDREN AND ADOLESCENTS

CBT for Depression in Children and Adolescents

A Guide to Relapse Prevention

Betsy D. Kennard
Jennifer L. Hughes
Aleksandra A. Foxwell

THE GUILFORD PRESS
New York   London

The authors have checked with sources believed to be reliable in their efforts to provide information that is complete and generally in accord with the standards of practice that are accepted at the time of publication. However, in view of the possibility of human error or changes in behavioral, mental health, or medical sciences, neither the authors, nor the editors and publisher, nor any other party who has been involved in the preparation or publication of this work warrants that the information contained herein is in every respect accurate or complete, and they are not responsible for any errors or omissions or the results obtained from the use of such information. Readers are encouraged to confirm the information contained in this book with other sources.

Library of Congress Cataloging-in-Publication Data

Names: Kennard, Betsy D., author. | Hughes, Jennifer L., 1981– , author. |
    Foxwell, Aleksandra A., author.
Title: CBT for depression in children and adolescents : a guide to relapse
    prevention / by Betsy D. Kennard, Jennifer L. Hughes, and Aleksandra A.
    Foxwell.
Description: New York: The Guilford Press, [2016]. | Includes
    bibliographical references and index.
Identifiers: LCCN 2015041065 | ISBN 9781462525256 (paper : alk. paper)
Subjects: | MESH: Child. | Cognitive Therapy—methods. | Adolescent. |
    Evidence-Based Medicine. | Secondary Prevention—methods.
Classification: LCC RJ505.C63 | NLM WS 350.2 | DDC 618.92/891425—dc23
LC record available at *http://lccn.loc.gov/2015041065*

About the Authors

Betsy D. Kennard, PsyD, ABPP, a clinical psychologist, is Professor in Psychiatry and Director of Cognitive-Behavioral Therapy (CBT) in the Pediatric Psychiatry Research Program at the University of Texas Southwestern Medical Center at Dallas (UT Southwestern) and Children's Health System of Texas. She also serves as Program Director of the Doctoral Program in Clinical Psychology at UT Southwestern and Clinical Director of the Suicide Prevention and Resilience Program at Children's Health. Dr. Kennard has been a site co-investigator on three multisite treatment studies of adolescent depression and suicide funded by the National Institute of Mental Health (NIMH) and has coauthored CBT treatment manuals for these studies. She developed this CBT sequential treatment strategy to prevent relapse in youth with depression and is currently Principal Investigator on an NIMH-funded treatment development study to treat suicidal adolescents.

Jennifer L. Hughes, PhD, is a clinical psychologist at Children's Health and Assistant Professor in Psychiatry at UT Southwestern. She has received funding from the American Foundation for Suicide Prevention to study an intervention designed to prevent future suicide attempts in youth, and she has served as a therapist, treatment developer, and co-investigator on several multisite studies of depressed and/or self-harming children and adolescents. Broadly, Dr. Hughes's research explores the efficacy and effectiveness of psychosocial approaches to the prevention and treatment of depression and suicide in youth and the dissemination of evidence-based treatments to the community.

Aleksandra A. Foxwell, PhD, is a clinical psychologist at the Student Wellness and Counseling Services and Assistant Professor in Psychiatry at UT Southwestern. She has served as a therapist and a co-investigator on several studies of suicidal children and adolescents with major depressive disorder. Dr. Foxwell's clinical interests focus on using evidence-based treatments for depression, anxiety, and other mood disorders in children, adolescents, and young adults. She also trains and supervises students and interns in using CBT for the treatment of depression.

Acknowledgments

First, we would like to thank the children and families who participated in the treatment studies of relapse prevention cognitive-behavioral therapy (RP-CBT). This work would not have been possible without their time, energy, effort, and input. Our work with them inspired many of the examples, as well as the fine-tuning of skills included in this book.

In addition, we are grateful to the National Institute of Mental Health (NIMH), who provided the funding for the clinical trials that led to the development of this treatment approach (NIMH R34 MH072737, principal investigator: B. Kennard; NIMH R01 MH39188, principal investigators: G. Emslie and B. Kennard).

We would like to acknowledge the original RP-CBT Development Team—Betsy D. Kennard, PsyD, Sunita Stewart, PhD, Jennifer L. Hughes, PhD, Puja Patel, PhD, Avery Hoenig, PhD, and Jessica Jones, MA—who were instrumental in developing the initial intervention. Additionally, we would like to thank Graham J. Emslie, MD, who was the co-principal investigator for the NIMH R01 randomized controlled trial to test RP-CBT. Given his experience in testing and developing continuation-phase treatments for youth depression, his input was invaluable in developing our approach to the clinical care of these children and their families.

We are also grateful to the many therapists, co-investigators, study coordinators, and graduate students who contributed to the success of this work: Taryn Mayes, MS, Jeanne Nightingale-Teresi, RN, MS, Carroll Hughes, PhD, RongRong Tao, MD, Kristi Baker, PhD, Mikah Smith, MA, LPC, Charlotte Haley, PhD, Kate Kennard, BA, Jessica King, BA, Alyssa Parker, PhD, Ashley Melson, MSW, Krystle Joyner, MS, Kristin Wolfe, MRC, Jarrette Moore, MA, Hayley Fournier, PhD,

Heather Lindburg, MS, Jeanne Rintelmann, BA, Lauren Smith, BA, Annie Walley, LCSW, Shauna Barnes, BA, and Tabatha Hines, PhD.

Thank you to Kevin Stark, PhD, and his graduate students, Kim Poling, MSW, John Curry, PhD, and Greg Clarke, PhD, for their careful review of the manual and helpful suggestions. In addition, we are grateful to those who served as consultants on the clinical trials of this manual, including David A. Brent, MD, A. John Rush, MD, Greg Clarke, PhD, Michael Frisch, PhD, Robin Jarrett, PhD, and Kevin Stark, PhD.

We would also like to acknowledge the influence of several important works that have shaped the development of RP-CBT. These individuals and their work have affected the care of depressed children and have had a major impact on our field.

1. *Treating depressed youth: Therapist manual for "ACTION."* (2007b). K. D. Stark, S. Schnoebelen, J. Simpson, J. Hargrave, J. Molnar, and R. Glen.

2. *Cognitive behavior therapy manual for TADS* (2000). J. Curry, K. Wells, D. Brent, G. Clarke, P. Rohde, A. M. Albano, M. Reinecke, N. Benazon, and J. March, with contributions by G. Ginsburg, A. Simons, B. D. Kennard, R. LaGrone, M. Sweeney, N. Feeny, and J. Kolker.

3. *Cognitive behavior therapy manual for TORDIA* (2000). D. Brent, M. Bridge, and C. Bonner.

4. *Cognitive therapy treatment manual for depressed and suicidal youth* (1997). D. Brent and K. Poling.

5. *Continuation therapy for major depressive disorder* (2001). R. B. Jarrett.

6. *Cognitive behavior therapy for suicide prevention (CBT-SP) teen manual, version 3* (2006). D. A. Brent, G. Brown, J. F. Curry, T. Goldstein, J. L. Hughes, B. D. Kennard, K. Poling, M. Scholossberg, B. Stanley, K. C. Wells, and the TASA CBT Team.

7. *The SAFETY Program: Ecological cognitive-behavioral intervention for adolescent suicide attempters* (2015). J. R. Asarnow, M. Berk, J. L. Hughes, and N. L. Anderson.

8. *Stress and your mood: Teen and young adult workbook* (1999). J. Asarnow, L. Jaycox, G. Clarke, P. Lewinsohn, H. Hops, and P. Rohde.

9. *Stress and your mood: A manual for individuals* (2010). J. Asarnow, L. Jaycox, G. Clarke, P. Lewinsohn, H. Hops, P. Rohde, and M. Rea.

For additional work related to RP-CBT, readers are referred to Kennard, Emslie, et al. (2008a); Kennard, Stewart, et al. (2008b); and Kennard et al. (2014).

Contents

CBT FOR DEPRESSION
IN CHILDREN AND ADOLESCENTS

CHAPTER 1

Introduction

MAJOR DEPRESSION IN CHILDREN AND ADOLESCENTS

An estimated 2% of children and 6% of adolescents suffer from depression, and the lifetime incidence is estimated at 4% for youth ages 3–17 (Perou et al., 2013; Birmaher et al., 2007), making this disorder a major public health concern. The lifetime prevalence of major depression in youth is estimated to be 20%, similar to adult populations (Birmaher, Arbelaez, & Brent, 2002). In addition, depressive disorders are a leading cause of morbidity and mortality in the pediatric age group (Birmaher et al., 2007). Depression is associated with decreased levels of functioning across domains, with higher severity associated with poorer functioning (Vitiello et al., 2006; Birmaher et al., 2004). Functional impairment in relationships, school, and the workplace, and frequent involvement in the legal system have been reported (Angold et al., 1998; Birmaher et al., 2007; Kandel & Davies, 1986; Kovacs et al., 1984a; Rohde, Lewinsohn, & Seeley, 1994). In addition, adolescents with depression are at increased risk for substance abuse, attempted and completed suicide, and recurrent depression in adulthood (Brent et al., 1988, 1993; Bridge, Goldstein, & Brent, 2006; Costello et al., 2002; Harrington, Fudge, Rutter, Pickles, & Hill, 1990; Kovacs et al., 1984b; Lewinsohn, Hops, Roberts, Seeley, & Andrews, 1993; Naicker, Galambos, Zeng, Senthilsevan, & Colman, 2013; Rao et al., 1995; Shaffer et al., 1996).

COURSE OF ILLNESS

Despite advances in acute treatment of pediatric depression, remission rates (defined as absence of symptoms; see definitions below) have been low. Even with the most comprehensive treatment (combination fluoxetine plus cognitive-behavioral therapy [CBT]) tested to date, only 37% of depressed adolescents remitted after 12 weeks of treatment in the Treatment for Adolescents with Depression Study (TADS; TADS Team, 2004). Additionally, residual symptoms are common following acute treatment. For example, in TADS (2004), 50% of acute treatment responders continued to have at least one residual symptom following acute treatment (Kennard et al., 2006). In addition, Tao, Mayes, Hughes, Rintelmann, and Emslie (2005) assessed residual symptoms in responders to open fluoxetine treatment, and found that even those youth with very few symptoms, considered to be in remission, continued to have residual symptoms (Tao et al., 2005). Residual symptoms are often associated with relapse and recurrence in adults (Fava, Fabbri, & Sonino, 2002; Karp et al., 2004; Montgomery, Doogan, & Burnside, 1991), and this appears to hold true for youth as well (Emslie et al., 2008).

As in adults, the course of illness in pediatric depression can be chronic. Although up to 90% of youth will recover within 1–2 years (Birmaher et al., 2002; Emslie et al., 1997b; McCauley et al., 1993; Strober, Lampert, Schmidt-Lackner, & Morell, 1993), relapse and recurrence rates are significant (Birmaher et al., 2002; Emslie et al., 1998; Lewinsohn, Allen, Seeley, & Gotlib, 1999; McCauley et al., 1993; Rao et al., 1995). Even of those youth who remain in treatment, 40% will relapse while on medication alone (Emslie et al., 2008). Much of the evidence to date suggests that once a youth has experienced a depressive episode, he or she is at a greater risk of developing a future episode (National Mental Health Association, 2004). As many as 50–75% of individuals with prepubertal major depressive disorder (MDD) have repeat episodes, spending 30% of their youth in an episode of depression (Emslie et al., 1997b; Kovacs et al., 1984b; Kovacs, Akiskal, Gatsonis, & Parrone, 1994; Lewinsohn et al., 1999; McCauley et al., 1993; Rao et al., 1995). Recurrence occurs most often during the 6 months to 1 year following remission (Emslie et al., 1998; Vostanis, Feehan, Grattan, & Bickerton, 1996; Wood, Harrington, & Moore, 1996). These life years, which are marked by disability, factor into the economic burden of the disease (Haby, Tonge, Littlefield, Carter, & Vos, 2004), with increased use of health care services and reduced productivity, costing tens of billions of dollars across the lifespan (Sturm & Wells, 1995). The combination of CBT and antidepressant medication has been shown to reduce health care costs over time (Domino et al., 2009).

DEFINITIONS OF OUTCOME

• *Response:* a significant reduction in major depressive symptoms for at least 2 weeks. In clinical trials, response is defined using a measure of clinical global improvement (CGI) or as changes in depressive symptom severity (e.g., 50% reduction in symptoms).

- *Remission:* minimal or no remaining depressive symptomatology, often defined in clinical trials using a cutoff on a clinical depression rating scale (e.g., Children's Depression Rating Scale—Revised [CDRS], scores ≤ 28).

- *Residual symptoms:* symptoms that remain after response to acute treatment.

- *Recovery:* no or minimal depressive symptoms of sufficient duration to be considered out of a depressive episode.

- *Clinical deterioration:* significant worsening so that treatment must be altered in order to prevent full relapse (Rush et al., 1998).

- *Relapse:* return of symptoms of the index episode (defined by a CDRS score of > 40 within a 2-week period or clinical deterioration).

- *Recurrence:* new episode of depression after recovery from the index episode.

CAN WE PREDICT REMISSION AND RELAPSE IN YOUTH?

It is important to be aware of factors that are related to the course of illness and treatment outcome. Although there is mixed evidence that demographic variables affect outcome, illness factors are predictive of course and treatment outcome. Factors such as severity of illness, comorbidity, recurrent depression, and insomnia are predictive of poorer outcome (Emslie, Mayes, Laptook, & Batt, 2003; Emslie et al., 2012). Similarly, psychosocial variables (e.g., parental psychopathology, family discord, and stressors) and history of trauma can predict poorer outcomes (Emslie et al., 2003; Kaufman et al., 2004; Nemeroff et al., 2003).

Few studies have examined predictors of relapse and recurrence. However, potential predictors include comorbidity (e.g., anxiety and behavior disorders, dysthymia), illness severity, recurrent depression, age of onset, suicidality, residual symptoms, poor functioning, insomnia, psychosocial stressors, family psychiatric history, and family discord (Birmaher et al., 1996a, 1996b, 2000; Emslie et al., 1997b, 1998, 2001; Klein, Lewinsohn, Seeley, & Rohde, 2001; Kovacs et al., 1984a; Lewinsohn et al., 1999; Rao, Hammen, & Daley, 1999; Weissman et al., 1999a, 1999b). Cognitive variables (e.g., hopelessness and ruminative thinking) may adversely affect treatment response and are associated with recurrent depression. Several studies report that negative cognitions are related to depression and may decrease with improvement in symptoms (Asarnow & Bates, 1988; Gotlib, Lewinsohn, Seeley, Rohde, & Redner, 1993; McCauley, Mitchell, Burke, & Moss, 1988; Tems, Stewart, Skinner, Hughes, & Emslie, 1993). Furthermore, dysfunctional thinking is a strong predictor of recurrent depression (Lewinsohn et al., 1999), and continued cognitive distortions following treatment may be predictive of shorter time to relapse (Beevers, Keitner, Ryan, & Miller, 2003).

DEFINITIONS OF TREATMENT PHASES

Treatment for MDD can be divided into three phases. The *acute phase* of treatment is designed to achieve symptom response (significant reduction in depressive symptoms) and ultimately remission (minimal to no symptoms). In clinical trials, the acute phase ranges from 6 to 12 weeks (Emslie et al., 2002, 2008; Kennard et al., 2014; TADS Team, 2004). Following acute treatment, the *continuation phase* of treatment targets residual symptoms to consolidate response and focuses on preventing relapse (defined as depressive episode after attaining remission). *Maintenance-phase* treatment, on the other hand, is a long-term treatment strategy designed to prevent new episodes, or recurrences, of depression in patients identified as having recovered from their index episode.

Acute-Phase Treatments

Antidepressant Medication

Acute-phase pharmacotherapy has been shown to be effective in the treatment of MDD in children and adolescents (e.g., Emslie et al., 1997a, 2002; TADS Team, 2004). Since the development of fluoxetine in 1988, selective serotonin reuptake inhibitors (SSRIs) and other newer antidepressants have been increasingly used to treat pediatric MDD (Cheung, Emslie, & Mayes, 2005). Other SSRIs, including citalopram, paroxetine, and sertraline, have also demonstrated some positive effect on at least some outcomes (Keller et al., 2001; Wagner et al., 2003, 2004), but only fluoxetine has been approved by the U.S. Food and Drug Administration (FDA) for treatment of child and adolescent depression and escitalopram, for the treatment of adolescent depression (Food and Drug Administration, 2014).

Promising Results: Acute-Phase CBT in Youth

A review of the literature in the area of acute treatment with CBT favors the effectiveness of this approach in both children and adolescents (Compton et al., 2004; Klein, Jacobs, & Reineke, 2007; Weisz, McCarty, & Valeri, 2006) over other psychosocial interventions or wait-list controls. CBT is a logical treatment to use as a psychosocial continuation-phase treatment, as other empirically tested psychotherapies (interpersonal therapy, systemic behavioral family therapy, and supportive therapy) have not been as well studied. See Table 1.1 for a review of acute-phase CBT trials.

Combination Treatment

TADS, a multisite trial sponsored by the National Institute of Mental Health (NIMH), compared fluoxetine, CBT, combination fluoxetine plus CBT, and placebo

TABLE 1.1. Acute-Phase CBT Trials

Trial (year)	Results
Asarnow et al. (2002)	CBT showed improvement in depression and negative thoughts over wait list.
Brent et al. (1997)	CBT showed more rapid remission in depression than family therapy and supportive therapy.
Brent et al. (2008)	CBT combined with a switch to medication showed a higher response rate than a medication switch alone.
Butler et al. (1980)	Role play and CBT showed more decrease in depression than wait list.
Clarke et al. (1999)	CBT groups led to higher recovery rates and decreased self-reported depression than wait list.
Kahn et al. (1990)	CBT showed reduced depression and reduced self-esteem compared to relaxation and self-modeling.
Lerner & Clum (1990)	CBT showed reduced depression, loneliness, and helplessness compared to supportive therapy.
Lewinsohn et al. (1990)	CBT groups were equally effective in treating depression and superior to waitlist.
Liddle & Spence (1990)	No difference was found between CBT, attention placebo, and no treatment.
March et al. (2004)	CBT alone had a higher rate of response than placebo, but lower than fluoxetine alone or fluoxetine with CBT.
Reynolds & Coats (1986)	Group CBT and relaxation were superior to wait-list control in reducing depressive symptoms.
Rosello & Bernal (1999)	CBT and IPT were more effective in treating MDD than wait list.
Stark et al. (1987)	CBT and self-control showed significant improvement over wait list.
TADS Team (2004)	Combination therapy was the most effective treatment for MDD. CBT was not superior to placebo.
Vostanis et al. (1996)	There was no difference between CBT and supportive therapy; both groups improved.
Weisz et al. (1997)	CBT showed greater reductions in depressive symptoms than control.
Wood et al. (1996)	CBT showed greater improvement in depression and overall outcome than relaxation therapy.

Note. CBT, cognitive-behavioral therapy; IPT, interpersonal therapy; MDD, major depressive disorder.

in 439 adolescents (ages 12–18). Acute response rates based on CGI ("very much" or "much" improved) were greatest for combination (71%), followed by fluoxetine alone (61%), CBT (43%), and placebo (35%). Both combination and fluoxetine alone were more effective than placebo, but CBT was not (TADS Team, 2004). While TADS demonstrated superiority for combination over medication alone for some outcomes, recent studies showed that fluoxetine plus CBT was not more effective than fluoxetine plus good clinical management (Clarke et al., 2005; Dubicka et al., 2010; Goodyer, 2006). Despite inconsistent outcomes, combination treatment is often considered the treatment of choice. However, when to initiate psychotherapy is less clear.

Continuation-Phase Treatment

Following successful acute treatment, adding CBT as a continuation-phase treatment of depression in adults has been found to produce reduced rates of relapse compared to placebo (Jarrett et al., 2013). In addition, adult studies indicate that relapse rates can be significantly reduced by augmenting psychopharmacotherapies with CBT in the continuation phase of treatment for major depression (Fava, Grandi, Zielezny, Canestrari, & Morphy, 1994; Fava, Grandi, Zielezny, Rafanelli, & Canestrari, 1996; Fava et al., 1998a, 2002, 2004; Guidi, Fava, Fava, & Papakostas, 2011; Nierenberg, 2001; Paykel et al., 1999; Paykel, 2007, Teasdale et al., 2000). Adult patients who have an adequate response to antidepressant medications continue to show a high rate of residual symptoms (in as many as 45% of these patients; Fava, Ottolini, & Ruini, 1999), as well as high rates of relapse (60% who have had one episode will have another).

In adult studies, CBT has been used to target residual symptoms and prevent relapse. Fava and colleagues (Fava et al., 1998a, 2004) have found that delivering CBT, which includes lifestyle modification training and well-being therapy after acute-phase treatment, is very effective in reducing symptoms and preventing relapse. In addition, given that the treatment was provided to remitted patients, who are therefore "less ill," the intervention could be administered in fewer sessions (10 every other week), as opposed to 16–20 (more typical in clinical trials of CBT). The cost effectiveness of continuation-phase CBT as a treatment strategy in reducing symptoms and preventing relapse has been documented (Scott, Palmer, Paykel, Teasdale, & Hayhurst, 2003).

Continuation-phase CBT after acute-phase pharmacotherapy, known as a sequential treatment strategy, has been shown to reduce both relapse and recurrence in adults (see Table 1.2). Although the treatment approach varied among the studies (e.g., well-being therapy, mindfulness), all studies used a CBT model.

There have been some recent efforts at health promotion or positive psychology that may inform the treatment of remitted youth. Ryff and Singer (1996) provide a model for defining dimensions of wellness in adults, which was later adapted into intervention strategies for relapse prevention in adults remitted for depression (Fava et al., 1998a). Seligman (Seligman & Csikszentmihalyi, 2000) and the movement of positive psychology emphasize the need for practitioners to focus more attention on amplifying strengths and building positive traits (e.g., optimism) as a means of preventing illness (Duckworth, Steen, & Seligman, 2005; Kobau et al., 2011).

Few studies have investigated relapse prevention strategies in youth. To date, there have been four trials in youth that employed a continuation-phase CBT intervention: one with positive results (Kroll, Harrington, Jayson, Fraser, & Gowers,

TABLE 1.2. Continuation- and Maintenance-Phase CBT in Adults

Trial(year)	Sample	Acute treatment	Length of acute treatment	Continuation-treatment arms	Outcome
Bockting et al. (2005)	N = 187 (recurrent MDD)	Not controlled; remission ≥ 10 weeks, but ≤ 2 years	Unknown	CT + TAU versus TAU (medications not controlled)	No difference between groups; CT + TAU had less relapse in patients with five or more episodes
Fava et al. (1994, 1996, 1998b)	N = 40	Antidepressant medication	12–20 weeks	CBT + MM (all medications tapered at start of continuation phase treatment)	Relapse at 2 years (15% vs. 35%); CBT + MM had greater reduction in residual symptoms
Jarrett et al. (2001)	N = 156	CT versus control	20 session	CT versus control	Continuation was shown to reduce rates of relapse
Paykel et al. (1999)	N = 158	Antidepressant	≥ 8 weeks	CBT + MM versus MM	Relapse (29% vs. 45%)
Perlis et al. (2002)	N = 132	Fluoxetine	8 weeks	CBT + MM versus MM	Relapse (6% vs. 8%)
Petersen et al. (2004)	N = 391	Fluoxetine	8 weeks	CBT + medications versus MM	No significant difference in HAMD-17 scores; CBT + medications had a more positive change in attribution style
Teasdale et al. (2000)	N = 145 (recurrent MDD)	Not controlled; (no medications past 12 weeks)	Unknown	MBCT versus TAU (medications not allowed)	No difference between treatments for two episodes; for three or more episodes: MBCT 40% versus TAU 66%

Note. CT, cognitive therapy; CBT, cognitive-behavioral therapy; HAMD-17, 17-item Hamilton Depression Rating Scale; MBCT, mindfulness-based cognitive therapy; MDD, major depressive disorder; MM, medical management; TAU, treatment as usual.

1996) and one with negative results (Clarke, Rohde, Lewinsohn, Hops, & Seeley, 1999). However, in both of these trials the acute phase of treatment was also CBT. In addition, in the negative trial, there was evidence that continuation-phase CBT was helpful to those who had not yet fully recovered at the end of acute treatment. In a pilot study, Kennard et al. (2008a), found risk of relapse to be eight times lower in youth ages 11–17 who were treated with a sequential treatment strategy. This pilot study was able to establish feasibility, acceptability, and preliminary efficacy of this continuation CBT approach (relapse prevention CBT [RP-CBT]) after response to acute antidepressant treatment. In a larger randomized controlled trial, these results were replicated with lower relapse rates over a 30-week treatment period in those treated openly with 6 weeks of antidepressant medication followed by RP-CBT compared to those treated with medication only (9% vs. 26.5%; Kennard et al., 2014). The study also concluded that those who were treated with CBT had a higher percentage of wellness time and required a lower antidepressant dose (Kennard et al., 2014).

This book details the treatment manual used in the above randomized control trials (Kennard et al., 2008a, 2014). The manual targets those who have had a favorable response to acute-phase treatment and was designed to be delivered in the continuation phase of treatment. In particular, our RP-CBT targets residual symptoms and teaches the child specific skills that will reduce these symptoms and prevent their recurrence. In addition, we have included wellness strategies and lifestyle changes designed to extend the period of recovery.

The treatment was designed to address risk factors that have been associated with relapse in children and adolescents, such as high expressed emotion and family conflict and disagreement (Asarnow, Goldstein, Tompson, & Guthrie, 1993; Birmaher et al., 2000). In addition, we find that certain cognitive factors have been linked to recurrence such as negative attributional style and cognitive reactivity (Hammen, 1992; Teasdale et al., 2001). Children who have had a depressive episode are at risk for reactivating negative schemas and negative attributions when faced with stress or change (positive or negative; Curry & Craighead, 1990). Therefore, the treatment is designed to counteract these negative schemas and attributions when the individual is faced with both positive outcomes and stressors (Jaycox, Reivich, Gillham, & Seligman, 1994; Seligman, Steen, Park, & Peterson, 2005). Finally, the treatment is meant to target residual symptoms of depression. Common residual symptoms in adults treated for depression include irritability, anxiety, and interpersonal friction (Fava et al., 1999), whereas common residual symptoms in adolescents treated for depression include sleep and mood disturbance, fatigue, and concentration difficulties (Kennard et al., 2006). Treatment components that address these residual symptoms are included in the manual as well as family interventions selected for the prevention of factors related to relapse (e.g., expressed emotion).

CHAPTER 2

Overview and Rationale

The overall goal of RP-CBT is to develop lifelong strategies to prevent depression and promote mental health. RP-CBT was specifically developed to improve acute- and continuation-phase treatment outcomes in youth with depression, employing a sequential treatment strategy in which patients are first treated with antidepressant medication (in particular, fluoxetine; Kennard et al., 2014). In line with the consensus recommendation definitions put forth by Frank and Kupfer (Frank, 1991; Kupfer, 1991), the goals of acute-phase treatment include clinical response and remission of symptoms. This phase typically lasts 6–12 weeks, and in RP-CBT the acute-phase treatment focuses on addressing residual symptoms to achieve remission and improved overall functioning. The goals of continuation-phase treatment include preventing relapse of symptoms of the treated episode. This phase can last up to 6–9 months (Birmaher et al., 2007; Emslie et al., 2008), and in RP-CBT the continuation-phase treatment focus is on both the prevention of relapse and recurrence of depression and the promotion of health and wellness. In summary, this treatment program was designed to increase the likelihood of remission, decrease residual symptoms, increase wellness, and reduce relapse.

RP-CBT was developed and tested within a sequential treatment strategy approach. The rationale for this approach is to improve clinical status (e.g., mood, concentration, energy) quickly through the use of antidepressant medication and then to optimize the treatment gains by introducing the psychosocial component when the youth is more likely to be receptive to the treatment owing to reduced depressive symptoms. In addition, the later introduction of the additional treatment can more specifically target residual symptoms, which are known to predict relapse.

Deferring psychotherapy may also allow for fewer sessions of more focused therapy. Even though the addition of CBT increases treatment costs, the utilization of short, intensive psychotherapy that prevents relapse and recurrence of depression is cost effective overall (Scott et al., 2003).

As a heuristic, we conceptualize acute-phase treatment as primarily returning the youth's mood to the baseline or neutral level. In contrast, in RP-CBT, which cuts across both the acute and continuation phases of treatment, we aim to not only work to improve the patient's mood to baseline but also to enhance mood above this neutral point. Treatment programs for acute-phase depression also include strategies to increase positive cognitions; however, the focus of these interventions is on mobilization against the behavioral and cognitive concomitants of depression. The early treatment response phase of depression is frequently marked by a significant decrease in negative cognitions, which offers the opportunity to provide preventive and enhancing strategies. The current treatment model shares some features with the acute treatment model (especially where the residual symptoms are more prominent), but also incorporates a qualitative shift to focus on strategies to promote enhancement above baseline of mood and activity. Thus, in this program we will conceptualize the youth's treatment not just from a deficit model (i.e., decreasing negative mood and cognitions), but also focusing on enhancement of strengths, positive experiences, mood, and cognitions. In summary, the treatment is driven by the goal to achieve the absence of illness and also the presence of wellness. The result is a two-prong treatment approach, including the following:

1. Skills that counter dysphoric mood and reduce stress (Brent, Bridge, & Bonner, 2000; Brent & Poling, 1997; Clarke et al., 1999; Curry et al., 2000; Fava et al., 1998a; Jarrett & Kraft, 1997; Stark et al., 2007a; Wilkes, Belsher, Rush, & Frank, 1994).

2. Strategies that promote health and well-being (mastery, positive self-regard, goal setting, quality relations/social problem solving, optimism; Jaycox et al., 1994; Ryff & Singer, 1996; Segal, Williams, & Teasdale, 2002; Seligman & Csikszentmihalyi, 2000; Snyder & Lopez, 2005) above the neutral level.

UNIQUE TREATMENT ELEMENTS OF RP-CBT

RP-CBT differs from typical acute CBT treatment programs for depression. The goal of acute CBT is to treat the current depressive episode, whereas the goal of RP-CBT is to treat the remaining symptoms of the episode and anticipate future challenges based on the patient's past experiences. Additionally, RP-CBT includes fewer core strategies, less "education," and more practice than traditional acute CBT approaches. The treatment is briefer and more focused as patients are already demonstrating treatment response when starting the program. Treatment is individually tailored, using core skills and supplements to address residual symptoms and relapse prevention risk. Other unique aspects of RP-CBT are summarized in the following sections.

Psychoeducation about Depression, Remission, and Relapse

Whereas many acute CBT programs include psychoeducation about depression, RP-CBT expands the education to include information about the episodic nature of depressive episodes, remission as the goal of treatment, and the risk of relapse and recurrent depression. To understand depressive symptom presentation, including the symptoms of the episode at its worst and any remaining residual symptoms, patients are encouraged to develop a timeline (discussed below). Additionally, therapists and patients can use assessment measures to track symptom severity and change over time, such as the Quick Inventory of Depressive Symptomatology—Self Report–16 (QIDS-SR-16; Rush et al., 2003), the Children's Depression Inventory–2 (CDI-2; Kovacs, 1992), or the Center for Epidemiologic Studies Depression Scale (CES-D; Radloff, 1977), among other self-reports of depressive symptoms. Youth are encouraged to develop their own ways of tracking mood, such as using mood diaries or mood-tracking phone applications. Patients are further educated about "lapse" versus "relapse" in an effort to help youth and families understand the need to track mood and symptoms over time and how to respond if symptoms are recognized.

This component promotes the belief that development of lifelong strategies and changes is important to preventing relapse and recurrence in those with a history of depression. A lifelong, lifestyle change is emphasized. Therapists introduce this idea by comparing the lifestyle changes to those changes required in individuals with cardiovascular disease: Following a heart attack, change is required for more than an "acute" phase of illness—with diet/exercise and other lifestyle changes necessary for wellness.

Timeline

At the beginning of RP-CBT treatment, a timeline is developed with the patient and family, which includes a review of the patient's past stressors, current residual symptoms, strengths and current skills, and treatment goals. A critical piece of the timeline is to help the patient identify potential challenges and obstacles that may trigger a relapse. The timeline serves as a conceptual model for treatment. Furthermore, with fewer sessions and longer gaps between meetings, the timeline fosters continuity and focus.

The timeline serves as a structure to individualize, plan, organize, and integrate the treatment. Throughout the treatment, the therapist and youth continue adding new skills, building strengths, identifying triggers, recognizing stressors, and proposing new ways to think about the self and the world. The timeline also references skills and wellness strategies.

The youth's timeline is collaboratively developed and guides the interventions. A handout assists the therapist in developing this timeline with the youth. Past stressors and symptoms, along with the youth's strengths and current skills, are outlined, as well as current (residual) symptoms/struggles, anticipated challenges, and obstacles ahead, along with the youth's goals and anticipated successes. In contrast to the acute phase when the focus is primarily in the present and the emphasis is on the rapid development of skills to actively reduce dysphoria, in the later phases it is important to integrate the past (acute depression and its symptoms) with a future-oriented outlook (i.e., prevention of future depression).

CBT Skills to Address Depression

Although the core skills in RP-CBT are not unique to this treatment, the selection of core skills and smaller scope of skills is unique to this briefer intervention. In RP-CBT, core skills for addressing depression and reducing stress include the following: behavioral coping skills (Stark, Reynolds, & Kaslow, 1987), cognitive restructuring (Brent et al., 1997), and problem solving (Butler, Meitzitis, Friedman, & Cole, 1980; Stark et al., 1987). Research shows that children who have had a depressive episode are at risk for reactivating negative schemas and negative attributions in the face of stress or change (positive or negative; Curry & Craighead, 1990). Therefore, in an effort to counteract these negative schemas and attributions, we will assess attributions and explanatory style when faced with both positive outcomes and stress. (Jaycox et al., 1994; Seligman, Schulman, DeRubeis, & Hollon, 1999). We found that having fewer core strategies results in more time for practice and integration of skills into the youth's life. Thus, the three core strategies—behavioral coping skills, automatic negative thoughts/cognitive restructuring, and problem solving—are taught and applied to the youth's residual symptoms and identified targets that might potentially lead to relapse. The practice of these skills between sessions is emphasized. In each session, a skill is applied to the youth's agenda, issues, timeline, treatment, and life goals. Again, the smaller number of sessions in RP-CBT makes a practical approach more important.

Core Beliefs ("Self-Beliefs"), Positive Self-Schema, and Attributional Style

RP-CBT emphasizes cognitive restructuring throughout the course of the program. Support for this particular approach has been recommended in youth (Brent et al., 1997; Bridge & Brent, 2004; Hollon et al., 2005). Even prior to the first session, the therapist formulates a draft conceptualization based on information from the earlier acute phase of medication treatment and self-report measures. This case conceptualization can be tested and expanded as the treatment process develops. In this program, the goal is to get to the core beliefs for each youth as early as possible (ideally in Session 1). This process includes educating the youth about core beliefs ("self-beliefs") and engaging the youth in testing these beliefs by gathering evidence (1) against the negative self-belief and (2) in favor or support of a positive self-schema (Beck, 1995). Typically, core beliefs fall into two categories: "I am helpless" and "I am unlovable" (Beck, 1995). In this program, we address three categories of self-belief: "I am inadequate," "I am worthless," and "I am unlovable" (K. Stark, personal communication, 2005). The idea of self-beliefs and building the positive self-schema is introduced in Sessions 1 and 2. Session 3 is exclusively devoted to core beliefs, self-schema, and cognitive restructuring.

RP-CBT includes an emphasis on attributions for positive events and works to build a positive self-schema and optimistic explanatory style. Although this is a common goal of traditional CBT approaches, in RP-CBT youth are better able to focus and integrate positive attributions as their depressive symptoms have slightly improved when starting the program (and with that, some of the more intense depressogenic thinking has also improved). Because youth struggling with depression tend to focus on negative outcomes, acute-phase treatment typically emphasizes the reduction of internal, stable, and global attributions for these outcomes. As mood and activation improve with the reduction of depressive symptoms, youth have more access to positive events, allowing therapists to highlight the cognitions related to these events. Relapse prevention is supported by questioning external and unstable attributions and promoting internal, stable explanations for such positive events.

Relapse Prevention and Wellness

Preventing relapse involves reducing negative factors thought to be related to depression and increasing positive factors found to promote well-being. Well-being can be defined as one's affective and cognitive assessment of the quality of life (Diener, 1984). There has been recent interest and growth in the area of positive psychology, or a focus on the building of positive experiences and individual traits (Seligman & Csikszentmihalyi, 2000). A meta-analysis of treatment studies using positive psychology interventions in both pediatric and adult populations shows promising results for the treatment of depression (Sin & Lyubomirsky, 2009). Based on Ryff and Singer's model (1996) on the development of psychological well-being, Fava and colleagues (1998b) applied wellness strategies to a clinical population of adults. These individuals had remitted for affective illness but continued to experience residual symptoms. In this study, results included decreased relapse rates and decreased symptoms in those who received cognitive behavioral and well-being therapy in the continuation phase of treatment. Fava based his well-being therapy on Ryff and Singer's six dimensions of wellness: self-acceptance, positive relations with others, autonomy, environmental mastery, purpose in life, and personal growth. Well-being therapy has been shown to prevent relapse in adults with affective illness. Similar work has been done with at-risk populations of children and young adults (Gilham et al., 2012; Jaycox et al., 1994; Seligman et al., 1999), focused on changing explanatory style and developing social problem-solving skills as a means of preventing future moderate depressive episodes.

In RP-CBT, we assess and build on the current wellness-related skills/strengths that the youth and family bring to the treatment. In particular, the RP-CBT program emphasizes strategies that promote health and wellness (adapted from Jaycox et al., 1994; Ryff & Singer, 1996; Seligman et al., 1999), coded as the six S's: (1) self-acceptance, (2) social, (3) success, (4) self-goals, (5) soothing, and (6) spiritual. Self-acceptance includes strategies to develop positive self-schema and a positive explanatory style. Social wellness includes a focus on planning and engaging in social activities, as well as enhanced social skills and social problem solving. The success component emphasizes autonomy and mastery, while the self-goals component focuses on purpose. The soothing component of wellness emphasizes planned relaxation and rest. Last, the spirituality component within our wellness program is broadly defined and individualized for each patient and may include meditation, altruism, gratitude, and values, as well as more traditional forms of spirituality such as religious beliefs (Pargament & Mahoney, 2005). RP-CBT is designed to identify the unique strengths, or in this case, the sources of spirituality that the patient already has, and to reinforce those aspects of spirituality already present in the patient. Although there are few empirical studies using spirituality in treatment, preliminary data from the field of positive psychology suggest that including this component can be an effective intervention (Frisch, 2006; McCullough, 1999; Propst, Ostrom, Watkins, Dean, & Mashburn, 1992).

RP-CBT TREATMENT

Structure and Sequence of Sessions

The primary interventions in RP-CBT are psychoeducation on relapse prevention, introduction and practice of skills to manage mood, identification of relapse factors with strategies specific to each factor, and development of wellness skills unique to each youth. Each child and family is provided with psychoeducation and skills selected for the individual child and family based on the assessment of relapse risk factors and appropriate wellness strategies, which are identified early in treatment (sessions one and two). Treatment also includes developing core behavior coping skills, managing automatic negative thoughts and cognitive restructuring, problem solving, and reducing negative emotion in the family. The practice of core skills and the application of these skills to individual issues are emphasized. Supplements, including emotional regulation, social skills, assertiveness training, and relaxation training and sleep hygiene, are included to assist the therapist in applying the core skills to these common issues encountered by youths. Other supplemental strategies include suggested strategies for common residual symptoms, such as boredom, anxiety, self-esteem issues, impulsivity, irritability, hopelessness, interpersonal conflict, and adherence. (In addition, guidelines for managing suicidality are included in the Appendix.)

STAGES OF TREATMENT

RP-CBT consists of three stages, which in the clinical trial took place over a 6-month period of time. The treatment was designed to be a brief therapy ranging from 8 to 11 sessions. In the randomized controlled trial of RP-CBT, the average number of sessions was nine (Kennard et al., 2014). However, the number of sessions can be individualized based on clinical need (i.e., those with more residual symptoms or greater severity; see Figure 4.1 in Chapter 4).

Stage 1

During the first 4 weeks of treatment, the youth and family attend weekly visits. Conjoint psychoeducation is conducted in Sessions 1 and 2. The objectives of this stage are to introduce core skills, assess and identify core beliefs, and identify and increase areas of strength and wellness for each youth (i.e., building a positive self-schema). Session 1 includes the assessment of target relapse factors, individual strengths, and treatment and personal goals (using a timeline of symptoms—past, present, and anticipated future problems), which is conducted in both an individual session and a conjoint session. In Session 2, the treatment plan is reviewed and refined (including skills identified for teaching), and we collaboratively develop treatment goals with the youth and family. Also in Session 2, behavioral coping skills and wellness training are introduced. In the conjoint session, psychoeducation on relapse prevention is reviewed, and skills to reduce family negative emotion are introduced. In Session 3, we assess skill acquisition from Session 2 and introduce managing automatic negative thoughts and cognitive restructuring (with emphasis on building a positive self-schema). Session 4 focuses on problem solving, the last "core skill." Each new skill is added to the timeline to demonstrate how the skill fits in with reducing depressive symptoms (past events on the timeline), maintaining gains, and managing mood (present and future).

Stage 2

This stage lasts 8 weeks, with four sessions of treatment (once every other week for 8 weeks). Sessions can be individual or family, with a minimum of one family session. Session 5 focuses on increasing strengths and developing wellness strategies. In Sessions 6 and 7, we emphasize practicing and applying the skills taught in the previous sessions, and we may include supplements to teach skills as needed, based on the target relapse factors. The content of sessions includes review and modification of relapse prevention strategies to target relapse risk factors. An ongoing review of symptoms and plans for managing residual symptoms are a priority of treatment at this stage (see the section on assessment). In Session 8, the therapist, youth, and family finalize the Relapse Prevention Plan and the Wellness Plan. Throughout the course of RP-CBT, all worksheets, Make It Stick Post-it notes, and postcards are kept. These are put in chronological order in a binder specific to each patient. The patient is provided with the binder to take home and a certificate at the end of this session.

Stage 3

This stage takes place over a 12-week period, with three optional booster sessions (which can be individual or family depending on the needs of the youth), with a suggested schedule of meeting once per month. The focus in this phase is on encouraging the independence of the patient to manage his or her own relapse risk factors and on providing the family with strategies to assist the patient. Therapists can use these sessions in a flexible manner. The primary goals are to evaluate the Relapse Prevention Plan and Wellness Plan. Additional skills may be taught as needed, but the focus is on use of the relapse prevention strategies developed in Stages 1 and 2 and modification of the relapse prevention plan as needed. This stage of treatment is directed toward maintaining wellness, anticipating obstacles to wellness, and using skills learned to combat these obstacles.

COMMON COMPONENTS OF ALL SESSIONS

All sessions include the following components:

1. Provide parents with a handout on today's topic while they wait.
2. Set the agenda; elicit the youth's concerns and prioritize topics to discuss.
3. Rate mood and review self-reports (looking for possible residual symptoms).
4. Review the previous session (Did It Stick?, elicit feedback and summary), including a review of homework/practice from previous session and a discussion of any adherence obstacles.
5. Provide psychoeducation and skill teaching.
6. Fit the skill to the timeline.
7. Make homework/practice assignment and adherence check.
8. Elicit feedback and Make It Stick (each child is given a Post-it note with a "take-home message" to put in his or her room).
9. Provide a brief check-in with parent.

CHAPTER 3

Assessing Clients and Planning Treatment

CLINICAL PRESENTATION OF DEPRESSION

The clinical presentation of depression is typically characterized by at least 2 weeks of persistent change in mood manifested by depressed or irritable mood and/or loss of interest. Other symptoms include a change in appetite, weight, or sleep, decreased concentration and energy, persistent guilt, low self-worth, and thoughts of death or suicidal ideation or attempts. Further, these symptoms represent a change in functioning and cause impairment in relationships or performance of activities (i.e., school, extracurricular activities) and are not attributable to substance use, use of medications, other psychiatric illness, bereavement, or medical illness (American Psychiatric Association, 2013; Birmaher et al., 2007). Although the symptoms of MDD in children and adolescents may be similar to those of adults, some differences can be attributed to the child's developmental stage (Birmaher et al., 1996a, 1996b; Fergusson, Horwood, Ridder, & Beautrais, 2005; Kaufman, Martin, King, & Charney, 2001; Klein, Dougherty, & Olino, 2005; Lewinsohn, Pettit, Joiner, & Seeley, 2003; Luby, Mrakotsky, Heffelfinger, Brown, & Spitznagel, 2004; Yorbik, Birmaher, Axelson, Williamson, & Ryan, 2004). Children and adolescents may present with irritability, low frustration tolerance, somatic complaints, and/or social withdrawal (Birmaher et al., 2007),

Several psychiatric disorders including anxiety, attention-deficit/hyperactivity disorder (ADHD), oppositional defiant disorder, pervasive developmental disorders, and substance abuse, as well as conditions such as bereavement and depressive reactions to stressors, can mimic depression or overlap with symptoms of depression

(Birmaher et al., 2007). Furthermore, medical conditions (e.g., hypothyroidism, mononucleosis, anemia, certain cancers, autoimmune diseases, premenstrual dysphoric disorder, and chronic fatigue syndrome) and certain medications (e.g., stimulants, corticosteroids, and contraceptives) can induce depressive-like symptoms, making the differential diagnosis more complicated (Birmaher et al., 2007).

Another consideration when diagnosing depression is differentiating between unipolar depression and a depressive phase of bipolar disorder. This may be challenging as children and adolescents are often experiencing their first episode of depression when they present for treatment. The presence of a strong family history of bipolar disorder and psychosis and a youth's history of medication-induced mania or hypomania may signify the development of bipolar disorder (Birmaher et al., 1996a, 1996b, 2007). It is therefore important to carefully assess any subtle symptoms of hypomania when evaluating children for depression.

Comorbid diagnoses are common in youth who have been diagnosed with depression, with 40 to 90% of them having a comorbid diagnosis and 50% having two or more comorbid diagnoses (Birmaher et al., 2007). The most frequent comorbid diagnoses are anxiety disorders, disruptive disorders, and ADHD. In the recent randomized controlled trial using RP-CBT, 22% of youth had a comorbid diagnosis of anxiety and 33% had disruptive disorders (Kennard et al., 2014). Additionally, in adolescents, substance use disorder is also a prevalent comorbid diagnosis (Birmaher et al., 2007).

ASSESSING DEPRESSION IN YOUTH

Depression in youth is assessed by using a comprehensive diagnostic evaluation. A semistructured interview, such as the Schedule for Affective Disorders and Schizophrenia for School-Age Children–Present and Lifetime version (K-SADS-PL; Kaufman et al., 1997), is a widely used tool in assessing psychiatric disorders in children. Clinicians should build rapport with the child and be attentive to any observable manifestation of depression such as irritability, decline in school performance, disruption in sleep, and withdrawal from pleasurable activities, for some children may have difficulties verbalizing their feelings or may deny symptoms of depression (Birmaher et al., 2007). The evaluation typically includes an interview with the child and parents or caregivers, as well as other informants such as teachers, physicians, or peers, when appropriate. The evaluation should be sensitive to the child's and family's ethnic and cultural background, for this may influence the presentation of illness and the course of treatment (Birmaher et al., 2007).

Critical elements in general assessment include course of illness, including number of episodes, severity, time frame of current episode and related symptoms, family history, and functional impairment. Assessment of current and past treatment and treatment response can further indicate the severity of illness and guide the clinician to appropriate treatment recommendations (i.e., in the case of treatment-resistant depression). Other stressors or vulnerabilities assessed during the initial evaluation could contribute to the current depressive episode or residual symptoms. Protective factors and family or peer support should also be assessed in order for the therapist to determine family involvement in treatment. The child's functioning can be assessed using several scales, including the Children's Global Assessment Scale (Shaffer et al., 1983).

When using RP-CBT with children and adolescents, it is also helpful for the therapist to assess for the following: (1) temperament; (2) level of cognitive development (e.g., concrete versus abstract thinking abilities); (3) presence of comorbidities (e.g., if a youth has ADHD, then a shorter session might be warranted); (4) parental level of involvement (e.g., chronological and developmental age of the child); and (5) prior treatment and/or familiarity with the RP-CBT concepts.

MEASUREMENT-BASED CARE AND SELF-REPORTS

Measurement-based care has been linked to improvement treatment outcomes in adult depression (Trivedi, 2009; Pence et al., 2012). Self-report measures of depression prior to each session are helpful in tracking symptom improvement, residual symptoms, and progress in treatment. Self-report scales often require less time and training, and youths may be more forthcoming (Cusin, Yang, Yeung, & Fava, 2009). This is also a way to populate the agenda for those who do not easily come in with issues to discuss. Scales can range from those that cover all diagnostic criteria for depression to more focused, symptom-specific measures.

Several evidence-based self-report measures are available for use in treatment. These particular measures have been used in our studies and clinics; however, they do not constitute a comprehensive list of the available measures for use. Clinicians should be flexible in their approach to measurement-based care and select those measures that are most helpful.

Examples of Symptom Severity and Diagnosis Measures

• The Quick Inventory of Depressive Symptomatology—Adolescent Version Self-Report (QIDS-A-SR-17; Rush et al. , 2003, 2006) is a reliable and valid 17-item self-report instrument intended to assess the severity of the nine core symptoms of depression. It was adapted from the original 16-item QIDS by adding a 17th item measuring irritability to reflect the disturbed mood diagnostic criteria in youth presenting as either sadness or irritability (American Psychiatric Association, 2000; Rush et al., 2003).

• The Beck Depression Inventory–II (BDI-II) is a 21-item scale that addresses all nine symptom criteria used to assess the severity of depression. It is normed on ages 13–80, with a sixth-grade reading level. It is relatively quick to administer (approximately 5 minutes) and has good validity and reliability (Beck, Steer, & Brown, 1996; Kumar, Steer, Teitelman, & Villacis, 2002). Similarly, the Children's Depression Inventory–2 (CDI-2) measures the severity of depression in children and adolescents ages 7–17 (Kovacs, 2010). It is available as a multirater assessment, including teachers, parents, and child self-reports.

• On the Mood and Feelings Questionnaire (MFQ-C and MFQ-P), the child (ages 7–18) or parent rates agreement with 33 (or 34, on the MFQ-P) depressive symptoms using a Likert scale (0 = not true, 1 = sometimes, 2 = true). The advantage of the MFQ-C and MFQ-P is that it provides the clinician equivalent child and parent measures for interrater comparisons. The MFQ-C and MFQ-P have been valid measures of clinical remission in other clinical trials of juvenile patients with depression (Kroll et al., 1996; Wood et al., 1996).

• The Center for Epidemiologic Studies Depression Scale (CES-D) is a brief 20-item measure that measures number, type, and duration of depressive symptoms. It is appropriate for youth ages 13–17 and requires approximately 10 minutes to complete. The CES-D is valid and reliable and has been normed across diverse ethnicities (Radloff, 1977; Morin, Moullec, Maiano, Layet, & Ninot, 2011).

• In busy clinic settings, the Patient Health Questionnaire (PHQ-9) is also a good option, as it is very brief, but specific and sensitive to depression symptoms (Kroenke, Spitzer, & Williams, 2001). It has been used primarily with adults in primary care settings; however, an adolescent version is available (PHQ-A; Johnson, Spitzer, Kroenke, & Williams, 2005).

Examples of Symptom-Focused and Functioning Measures

Symptom-specific measures can also be a useful tool in treatment, specifically when addressing residual symptoms. We list several assessment tools that we have used in our clinical trials or outpatient clinics; however, the therapist should choose measures based on the patient's needs. These can range from cognitive scales to assessment of suicidal behaviors to overall functioning.

• The Cognitive Triad Inventory for Children (CTI-C; Kaslow, Stark, Printz, Livingston, & Tsai, 1992) is a revision of the CTI specific for school-age children (ages 6–18). This 36-item measure has shown good reliability and validity and includes three scales: view of the self, view of the world, and view of the future.

• The Children's Cognitive Style Questionnaire (CCSQ; Abela, 2001) consists of four negative and two positive scenarios, accompanied by statements regarding the internality, stability, and globality of attributions (three items per scenario). The patient indicates agreement with each item on a 5-point scale. This scale was designed for use with ages 6–18.

• The Hopelessness Scale for Children and the Hopelessness Scale for Adolescents (HSC and HSA; Kazdin, French, Unis, Esveldt-Dawson, & Sherick, 1983) are adapted from the Beck Hopelessness Scale (BHS; Beck, Weissman, Lester, & Trexler, 1974). The HSC is for use with children ages 6–11, and the HSA for ages 12–18. These measures have been shown to predict treatment response and dropout from treatment (Brent et al., 1999).

• The Columbia Suicide Severity Rating Scale (C-SSRS; Posner et al., 2008) was designed to measure four constructs: severity of ideation, intensity of ideation, suicidal behavior, and lethality with high sensitivity and specificity for classification of suicidal behaviors (Posner et al., 2011).

• The Multidimensional Students' Life Satisfaction Scale (MSLSS; Huebner, 1994) is a 40-item self-report scale for ages 7 and up designed to measure life satisfaction in youth. The MSLSS measures five domains—friends, family, school, self, and living environment—along with general life satisfaction. Patients rate their satisfaction across each area using four options (never, sometimes, often, almost always). Research has indicated acceptable psychometric properties for the MSLSS (Gilman, Huebner, & Laughlin, 2000).

TIMELINE AND ONGOING ASSESSMENT IN TREATMENT

In contrast to acute-phase treatment, where the focus is primarily on the rapid development of skills, the emphasis once a patient has achieved remission or response is integrating the past (acute depression and its symptoms) and preventing future depression. In RP-CBT the patient and therapist collaboratively build a timeline that will guide the intervention. The timeline is a detailed structured assessment of stressors, residual symptoms, triggers, and unhelpful thoughts (see Handout 3.1, My Timeline*). This helps the therapist individualize, plan, organize, and integrate the treatment. Typically, the timeline is done at the beginning of treatment and is modified as new skills are acquired.

At the beginning of treatment, the therapist uses the timeline to help identify residual symptoms as well as the youth's strengths. Throughout the treatment, the therapist and patient continue adding new skills, building strengths, identifying triggers, recognizing stressors, and devising new ways to think about the self and the world. Identifying goals and wellness strategies are referenced in the timeline.

---

*All patient handouts are at the ends of the respective chapters.

Because of the smaller number of sessions and longer gaps between meetings, the timeline is used to foster continuity and focus.

In addition to the timeline, the therapist also utilizes symptom monitoring throughout the treatment. The teen begins to monitor his or her mood at the onset of treatment using a mood monitor chart as well as an emotions thermometer. Mood monitoring is used as a scale to allow the patient to recognize his or her mood state and utilize skills learned in therapy. Various methods of mood monitoring are presented in the treatment manual. Other ongoing assessments may include tracking of undesirable behaviors such as isolating, engaging in substance use, and eating-disordered behaviors. As the patient progresses throughout the treatment, activity tracking and thought records are used to measure the use of behavioral coping strategies and unhelpful thinking.

MY TIMELINE

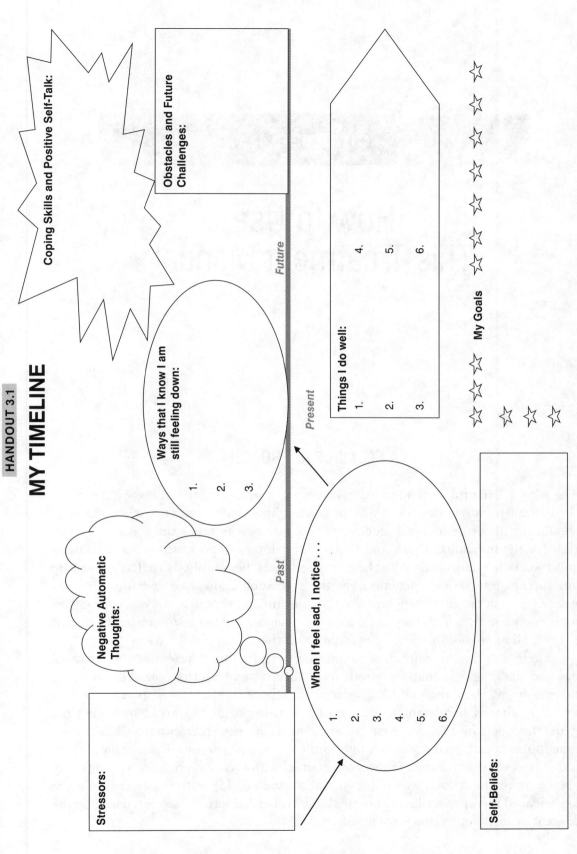

Coping Skills and Positive Self-Talk:

Obstacles and Future Challenges:

Negative Automatic Thoughts:

Ways that I know I am still feeling down:

1.
2.
3.

Stressors:

When I feel sad, I notice . . .

1.
2.
3.
4.
5.
6.

Things I do well:

1.
2.
3.
4.
5.
6.

My Goals

Self-Beliefs:

Past   Present   Future

CHAPTER 4

How to Use
This Treatment Manual

A FLEXIBLE APPROACH

The RP-CBT treatment is intended to be used in a *flexible* manner. It should provide the therapist with guidelines to use for content and session structure. The therapist should use his or her clinical judgment as to how best to tailor the skills and materials for the individual youth and family. Of primary importance is maintaining a good working relationship with the youth and his or her family, as well as addressing any therapy-interfering behaviors. The therapist should always do what is clinically necessary to maintain the therapeutic relationship and should address any problems with compliance, which may include some deviations from the manual. However, the overall approach should be consistent with the principles of CBT.

Therapists should maintain a balance between teaching the skills from the manual and making sure that the youth feels "heard" and understood. The therapist takes time to elicit the youth's concerns (collaboratively creating an agenda that includes what is important to the youth). It is important to avoid following the manual session by session (often an error made by new therapists) and failing to take into account what the youth put on the agenda or what went on in the youth's life that week. If a therapist follows the manual with too much rigidity, sessions may appear more like school, which does not allow for a collaborative approach. A more experienced therapist will incorporate the skills needed into the session based on the content of the youth's concerns/agenda.

We suggest the session order presented next because it is based on an ideal course of treatment. The therapist may vary this order according to the clinical needs of the patient and families.

- *Session 1: CBT and Relapse Prevention Program Overview/Rationale, and Establishing Timeline and Goals.* Education on relapse of MDD, risk factors for relapse, and wellness and well-being. In addition, mood monitoring and management are presented during psychoeducation.

- *Session 2: Behavioral Coping Skills and Family Expressed Emotion.* Teaching behavioral coping skills for managing mood and reducing negative emotion in the family.

- *Session 3: Cognitive Restructuring and Identifying Unhelpful Thoughts.* Teaching about the connection between thinking, mood, and behavior; distinguishing between thoughts that are "helpful" versus "unhelpful."

- *Session 4: Problem Solving.* Teaching problem-solving steps using the FLIP method.

- *Session 5: Identifying Skills for Maintaining Wellness and Building the Wellness Plan.* Developing wellness skills for the individual and family. Wellness strategies include lifestyle (behavioral) modifications and well-being therapy strategies addressing beliefs and attitudes.

- *Sessions 6 and 7: Practice and Application of Core Skills.* Reviewing core skills with the addition of optional supplements as needed.

- *Session 8: Relapse Prevention Plan and Wellness Plan.* Specifically using the timeline and skills learned to create the Relapse Prevention and Wellness Plan.

- *Sessions 9–11 (monthly for 3 months): Graduation Session and Booster Sessions.* Reviewing core skills and modifying the Relapse Prevention Plan and Wellness Plan as needed.

Note that supplemental materials to target relapse risk factors have been included in the Appendix. These materials are intended to be used according to patient need in order to assist the youth in applying the core skills to specific areas. Supplements include Adherence, Anxiety, Assertiveness, Anhedonia, Boredom, Emotion Regulation, Hopelessness, Impulsivity, Interpersonal Conflict, Irritability, Peer Victimization (Dealing with Bullies), Relaxation Training and Sleep Hygiene, Self-Esteem, Social Skills, Social Support, and Suicidality: Guidelines for Management. The order of sessions may vary depending on the youth's residual symptom profile (i.e., readiness for core skills versus wellness skills). See Figure 4.1 for a decision tree to guide the therapist in treatment planning.

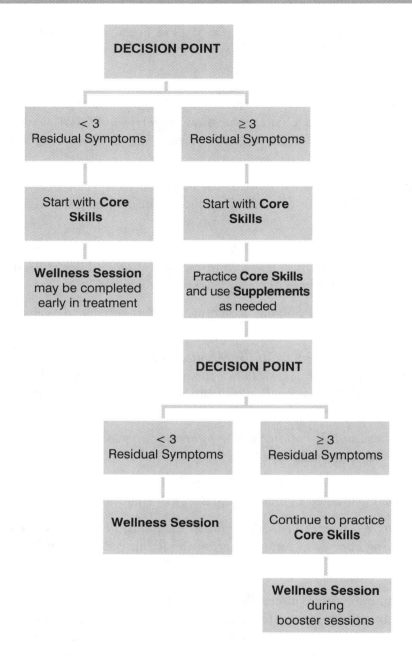

FIGURE 4.1. Decision tree for treatment planning.

THERAPIST STYLE

This manual was written with the awareness that each therapist has his or her own style of conducting therapy sessions. We have tried to accommodate these styles by including both specific suggested language and outlines to aid in structuring sessions and teaching skills. Therapists should feel comfortable adapting the language, as well as the suggested activities, according to their personal styles and the individual needs of the youth. Below is a stylistic guide to help the therapist understand the format of this treatment manual.

Italics	*Suggested language*
Shaded boxes	Tips for therapists
Boxes	In-session activities; suggested handouts

DEVELOPMENTAL CONSIDERATIONS

In this treatment, we will allow for developmental differences. The treatment will be modified for younger (or cognitively less mature) patients in the following wavys: (1) there will be more of a behavioral component to the treatment, (2) there will be more emphasis on role play in the session, and (3) there will be a greater use of visual materials versus more language-oriented materials. In addition, each session will include a parent component, or parent check-in, in which skills will be reviewed (in most cases with the child teaching the skill) with the parent. Parent participation in the relapse plan and any homework will be an important part of all child sessions.

ADDRESSING DIVERSITY

Sensitivity to issues of diversity is an important consideration for any therapist. Of note, in the randomized controlled trial of RP-CBT, 82% of participants identified their race as Caucasian and 30% identified their ethnicity as Hispanic (Kennard et al., 2014). Therapists using RP-CBT are asked to review the American Psychological Association *Guidelines for Providers of Psychological Services to Ethnic, Linguistic, and Culturally Diverse Populations* (available at *www.apa.org/pi/oema/resources/policy/provider-guidelines.aspx*). It is recommended that consultation be obtained when working with patients and families from different cultures and ethnic backgrounds.

SESSION CONTENT

Objectives and therapist checklists are provided for each session for easy reference. The first five sessions focus on the development of core skills. Additional supplements can be used during these sessions or in Sessions 6 and 7; *however, the primary focus should always be on core skills and self-beliefs* (i.e., always tie the supplement skills back to behavioral coping skills, cognitive restructuring, problem solving, and self-beliefs). Supplements may be used at any point during the treatment to address specific concerns of the youth or therapist. These supplements consist of skills that we anticipate will be needed by some youths (based on current residual symptoms or past symptoms of depression in the acute phase) to prevent relapse (Asarnow & Horton, 1990; Asarnow et al., 1993; Birmaher et al., 2000; Teasdale et al., 2001). Suggested handouts are included for each supplement.

The sessions include the following components or guides for the therapist:

- *Use This Core Skill for . . .* This section gives therapists tips to consider when planning treatment for a youth. These suggestions are meant to guide the therapist in deciding if a skill is appropriate for a youth.

- *Session Objectives.* Goals are listed for each session.

- *Session Checklist.* A checklist, uniform across most of the sessions, accompanies each session, which includes areas to cover at each visit (e.g., mood check, homework review). This checklist serves as the therapist's reminder to work within the CBT model or stick with the "the basics" of CBT (i.e., setting an agenda, monitoring mood).

- *Introduction.* Each session begins with a suggested introduction that includes ways for the therapist to introduce the new skill (suggested segues and language).

- *Rationale.* The rationale provides an explanation for the therapist and youth of the importance of the skill (i.e., why the skill is necessary or useful).

- *Teach.* This section provides the therapist with ideas about how to convey the skill to the youth. Suggested activities are included, and suggested handouts are referenced.

- *Practice in Session.* The therapist is provided with guidelines for practicing the skill with the youth either through *in vivo* experiences or through planning and role-playing a possible scenario where the skill could be used.

- *Apply to Timeline.* The therapist is given reminders to connect the skill (including any new strengths discovered) to the youth's timeline.

- *Homework/Practice.* The therapist and the youth should collaborate to identify how the youth can use what was learned in this session over the next week. Be specific! Suggestions are included for each skill.

- *Make It Stick*. This is one way to "cement" the skill or strategy for the youth. Have the youth share what he or she learned in the session and list these items on a Make It Stick Post-it note. The therapist can add any additional points to this list. The youth may also give feedback about what he or she found to be the most helpful from the session.

- *"Ideas for the Therapist"* box. Techniques for tailoring the session for developmentally less mature youth, as well as older youth, are included in each session.

- *Did It Stick?* These are suggested questions to begin the next session in order to assess if the youth understood the material that was covered previously.

The supplements are designed as follows:

- *Use This Supplement for . . .* This section gives therapists tips to consider when planning treatment for a youth. These suggestions are meant to guide the therapist in deciding if a skill is appropriate for a youth.

- *Skills to Consider*. Suggested core skills or additional supplements to use in conjunction with the supplement are listed.

- *Strategies to Try*. Strategies are suggested for teaching the youth to manage a particular issue or problem.

- *Suggested Handouts*. Suggested handouts to use with the supplement are referenced.

HOMEWORK/PRACTICE

The development of a homework assignment is an integral part of each session, as this encourages the youth to practice the skill(s) during the upcoming week. When assigning the homework, the therapist should elicit how likely the youth is to actually complete the homework (Adherence Check on a scale of 1–10). Then the therapist and youth should brainstorm ways to get that number as close to 10 as possible. Important factors to consider when assigning homework include:

1. Review the Rationale/Goals.
   - Tie homework to the timeline and relapse prevention plan.
   - Make homework relevant to the youth's goals.
2. Collaborate with the youth to create the homework assignment.
3. Confirm that the youth understands the instructions/homework assignment.

4. Investigate possible barriers to keep the youth from completing homework.
   • Rate the likelihood that homework will be done as assigned.
5. Practice homework in session.

As the sessions become less frequent, it may be necessary for the therapist and youth to brainstorm ways to help the youth remember the skills and the homework assignment. Suggestions include:

1. The therapist can mail the youth a reminder postcard during the week.
2. The therapist can send the youth a reminder email or text message.
3. The youth can ask the therapist to do a phone check-in between sessions for a memory boost.

MAKE IT STICK AND DID IT STICK?

Each session should end with a Make It Stick exercise. During this section of the session, the therapist should elicit feedback from the youth about the session (i.e., what was particularly helpful or unhelpful?). Have the youth share what he or she learned in the session and list these items on a Make It Stick Post-it note. The therapist can add any additional points to this list. Each session should also end with a Did It Stick? review to assess whether the youth understood and used the skill from the previous session. Questions have been included at the end of each session to help therapists to complete this knowledge check in the next session.

In the following chapters, we present the guidelines for each session, including session goals, content, suggested language, and handouts.

CHAPTER 5

Session 1

CBT and Relapse Prevention Program Overview/Rationale, and Establishing Timeline and Goals

Use This Core Skill for . . .

- All youth and parents to begin the relapse prevention program.

Session Objectives

- Build rapport with the youth and family.
- Introduce the youth to CBT and the relapse prevention rationale.
- Introduce the youth to collaboration, confidentiality, compliance, and communication.
- Identify the residual symptoms of depression.
- Begin timeline development.
- Assess the youth's attributions for positive outcomes/negative outcomes.

Session Checklist

1. Provide the parents with a handout on today's topic while they wait.
2. Set the agenda; elicit the youth's issues.
3. Introduce the CBT model and the relapse prevention rationale.
4. Begin timeline development and assessment of strengths and treatment goals.

5. Start this week's practice.

6. Elicit feedback and Make It Stick.

In this session, the first 45 minutes of treatment will be spent with the youth in an individual session, followed by a 45-minute conjoint session with the youth and parents. Prior to the session, you may begin a draft case conceptualization (including a hypothesis about the self-belief) using self-reports or information from clinical interviews.

INTRODUCTION

The primary goal of this session is to build rapport with the youth, while getting his or her "story" about past depression, present problems (residual symptoms), and future concerns. You should also introduce the CBT model, the relapse prevention program rationale, and therapy guidelines.

> **THERAPIST TIP:** Building rapport is of *utmost* importance in this session. If you do not get to everything, that is okay! Make sure to take time to really hear what the youth has to say! Be mindful not to "pull the bus out of the parking lot" without the youth on board (K. Poling, personal communication, 2005).

RATIONALE

Introductions

Begin this session by introducing yourself and your role with the treatment team (emphasizing the connection with the acute-phase team). Explain that you have reviewed their information from the acute phase of treatment and the assessments from the baseline of this continuation-phase treatment. It will be important to acknowledge the time and effort that they have put into their treatment up to this point and to get their thoughts and feelings about the progress they have made so far.

Taking Care of Business

Get the youth into the habit of beginning the session with an agenda and a review of self-reports. Therapy guidelines and expectations will be discussed later in this session. Beginning with an agenda for this session will help to introduce the structure to the youth, as well as communicate the importance of their agenda items in this treatment.

Agenda

Ask for any concerns or issues that the youth would like to include. Then explain what you hope to accomplish during the session (i.e., what the youth can expect). Orient the youth to the collaborative nature of agenda setting. Remember, you will want to elicit the youth's agenda at every session.

Suggested therapist-initiated agenda items for the first session include reviewing residual symptoms of depression, creating the timeline, and talking about treatment goals.

Mood Check/Symptom Review

Also go over self-reports at this time; future sessions should include a mood check (self-mood rating) and symptom review.

Brief Rationale for Treatment (Will Be Discussed Later during the Conjoint Session)

Rationale for the Treatment Model

Introduce the CBT treatment model. In addition, introduce the main themes and components of this treatment using Handout 5.3, My Relapse Prevention and Wellness Program.

- There are three parts of the self; each part influences the other parts.
- Provide an example to demonstrate the connection of each part of the self-triangle. Emphasize the reciprocal influence of the self-triangle. Each part of the triangle affects the other parts.

> ### *Sports Example*
> *"Edward, a beginning basketball player, is practicing his free throws. He begins missing his shots. He <u>thinks</u> to himself, 'I am terrible at basketball; I am awful; I will never be able to master this sport.' He decides to end his practice early, and practices less (<u>behavior</u>)—as a result, he begins to miss more shots on the next practice. More negative thinking, less active behavior, as a result, the mood drops. Do you see a cycle here?"*

> ### *Academic Example*
> *"Lucy is studying for a test. She begins to <u>think</u>, 'I will not pass this test; what's the point?' (Thinking is rather hopeless, right?) What happens to her <u>behavior</u>? She studies less, right? What are the chances that she will do well on the test without studying? How*

does her thinking affect her behavior? How can both thinking and behavior affect mood?"

Social Example

"Tina does not have a date for homecoming. She begins to <u>think</u>, 'No one will talk to me or hang out with me at the dance.' She goes to the dance but does not talk with anyone at the dance (<u>behavior</u>). What does Tina's thinking and behavior here do to her mood?"

- Elicit feedback from the youth (and parents) about the triangle. Ask if the youth notices the relationship between thoughts, behaviors, and feelings in his or her own life. What examples can he or she share with you?

- Introduce the concept of a scientific model testing thoughts and behaviors. Introduce the idea of skills/tools to the youth. Share how certain skills are especially useful to help "fight depression" (i.e., decrease certain symptoms or problems). Reinforce this idea by showing the youth Handout 5.3, My Relapse Prevention and Wellness Program, which lists each skill and what it will help with.

SUGGESTED HANDOUTS

✓ Self-Triangle (Handout 5.1)

✓ Mood Monitor Log (Handout 5.2)

✓ My Relapse Prevention and Wellness Program (Handout 5.3)

Rationale for the Program

The rationale is to prevent relapse of depressive symptoms. Provide education on relapse, and on lapse versus relapse. Reinforce and validate that the youth has skills that he or she is already using; we will build upon these skills. In addition, we will be looking back at past problems and anticipating future problems in order to determine what new skills might be helpful to the youth and to develop a Relapse Prevention and Wellness Plan.

THERAPIST TIP: You will want to *elicit the youth's thoughts and feelings about being in a continuation-phase* treatment (i.e., receiving treatment when not feeling particularly depressed).

TEACH

Therapy Guidelines

Introduce the "four C's": collaboration, communication, confidentiality, and compliance. Discuss the attendance and involvement of parents.

Collaboration

Discuss any prior psychotherapy experiences, highlighting the unique qualities of CBT (collaborative, active/homework, emphasis on thoughts/behaviors). Emphasize a team approach to therapy (e.g., agenda setting). Stress the importance of the youth "bringing something to the table."

Communication

Stress the importance of communication in therapy. Reinforce that you will use feedback (about what is helpful and not so helpful) to make changes accordingly. Ask the youth about the session up to this point to reinforce this idea.

> *"There will be times when I misunderstand you, or when the program seems not helpful or like it is taking up too much of your time. I hope you will let me know so that we can look at the situation together and decide how to make changes so that you get what you need."*

Confidentiality

Explain to the youth that the information that they share with you will be confidential, but discuss the limits of confidentiality. You will need to talk with their parents/caretakers in the event that they are in danger, or are in any way unsafe. However, if possible, you and the youth will discuss specific confidentiality issues in therapy and you will work with the youth to come to a decision about what to say and when and how to say it. Confidentiality may be compromised if any youth is in danger of hurting him- or herself (e.g., dangerous drug use, etc.) or others.

> *"What is your understanding of confidentiality?"*

Compliance

Introduce the concept of therapy homework (or "practice assignments")—collaborative assignments designed to help the youth practice the newly acquired skills. A challenge to any therapy program is the application of the skills outside of the session. Remind the youth that you will only spend an hour or so a week with him or her for 4 weeks, and then every other week after that. For it to work, relapse prevention is something that must be done daily, not just in sessions.

Attendance

Discuss the importance of attendance and any procedures for canceling or rescheduling appointments. Ask the youth if he or she anticipates any barriers to attendance.

> *"What are some obstacles that could keep you from coming for therapy? Let's just get those out in the open, and maybe we can be hands-on about it and come up with ways to avoid those now."*

Involvement of Parents

Explain the rationale for inviting parents to come in and what will be covered in the sessions. Elicit any concerns about this. Give time for discussion if including parents is an issue, and collaborate with the youth on how the parents will be involved. Involvement of parents is necessary, as having the proper support and reducing stress are essential to preventing relapse. A team approach can be helpful. Parents will be informed of skills, and the therapist will look for ways parents can help by reducing stress and conflict in the home, and increasing support for the youth.

SUGGESTED HANDOUT
✓ Expectations (Handout 5.4)

Getting the Story (Timeline): Developing a List of Residual Symptoms of Depression and Symptom Picture Prior to Acute Treatment

The main focus of this session is on *building rapport* with the youth. Remember, the youth may have already told this story to other health professionals or members of the treatment team, and you probably have had access to this information; remind the youth that it is good for you to hear it in his or her own words, so that you "won't miss anything."

- Get a sense of "the youth's story" on depression. Remember to be listening for any strong positive or negative self-beliefs.
- Can the youth tell you how he or she got into this treatment?
- For younger kids, it might be good to try the metaphor of a story, with a beginning, middle, and end:

"What happened before you got to treatment, and what has been happening lately in regard to your mood? Where are you now in the story? How would you like to write the next chapter of the story?"

- This is a good time to assess for any history of suicidal ideation (check for current as well) for the youth. Reassure the youth that this is common when one feels depressed. Also, inform the youth you will ask about this again in the future, especially if you have any reason to worry about his or her safety.

"At your very worst, did you ever feel like you wished you weren't here anymore, or that you wanted to harm yourself? Have you ever tried to hurt yourself in any way?"

THERAPIST TIP: Be sensitive to the youth's wishes to not want to go too much into talking about when he or she was depressed; however, explain that some information about how and why he or she got depressed (from the youth's point of view) will influence how we design a treatment program for him or her to defend against relapse. Remember, as well, that a mood and suicide check is important at every session; checking in on this "normalizes" the discussion!

REQUIRED ACTIVITY: **Timeline Development (This May Be Continued in Session 2)**

For this activity, you will need Handout 5.5, My Timeline. This handout enables you to show the youth how "old" symptoms from when he or she was depressed may be residual symptoms now. This handout also contains a place to list negative thoughts and new skills that the youth will eventually add as part of the Relapse Prevention Plan. Collaborate with the youth to begin to create the timeline based on the information provided by the youth.

"Depression is different for everyone. Remember back to when you were depressed, what did the depression 'look like' for you? How were you affected by it? How would I have known you were depressed? What does the depression look like today? What remains?

"What is likely to be a problem for you in the future? What are the things that may bring it back?"

You may also find it useful to review any self-report measures, diagnostic instruments, and/or clinical notes to help gain a better understanding of the youth's depression symptoms and difficulties over time.

For younger youth, Handout 5.6, Depression Pie, might be especially helpful. Ask the youth to identify the slices in his or her pie (What were the factors related to his or her depression? How big was each?). Give the youth an opportunity to look at a sample pie of depression. Can he or she create one that reflects his or her own experience?

Treatment Goals

Begin discussion of treatment goals. This is a good homework assignment to give for Session 1.

> SUGGESTED HANDOUT
> ✓ My Goals (Handout 5.7)

PRACTICE IN SESSION

Assess understanding of program/get feedback. Elicit feedback from the youth about the session and answer any remaining questions.
  Have the youth summarize the session for you.

"What was the main take-home message today?"

HOMEWORK/PRACTICE

Collaborate with the youth to identify how he or she can use what was learned in this session over the next week. Be specific!

Suggested Homework

Contract with the youth to review psychoeducational materials. Discuss with him or her the importance of understanding depression, in order to make a better relapse plan and to get the most out of the treatment. Assess with the youth the likelihood that he or she will read the psychoeducational materials. Identify any barriers or obstacles to completing this task and help to find solutions. For example, these may be viewed prior to the next session on site if needed.

> SUGGESTED HANDOUT
> ✓ The Basics of Depression (Handout 5.8)

Brainstorm ways to overcome any barriers or obstacles to completing the homework. Would a between-session postcard, email, text message, or phone call be helpful? Suggestions include:

1. Collaborate to review the psychoeducational materials.
2. Discuss with the teen his or her thoughts about completing Handout 5.7, My Goals, and return to discuss next week.
3. Provide the rationale and discuss with the youth his or her response to completing a Mood Monitor Log (Handout 5.2) over the following week.

MAKE IT STICK

Have the youth share what he or she learned in the session and list these observations on a Make It Stick Post-it note. Add any additional points to this list. The youth may also give feedback about what was the most helpful from the session. Share what you learned about the youth during this session (i.e., reinforce the youth's strengths).

- In this first session, inform the youth that Did It Stick? will occur in every session to review the previous week.
- In addition, you may create a postcard (or text message) to send the youth during the week with the main points from the session. This should help the youth remember to practice what was learned in session.

Suggested items for the Make It Stick include:

- Four C's of therapy.
- Reminder for the youth to review psychoeducational materials and complete any other homework or practice agreed upon.
- Treatment goals.
- Self-beliefs (if discussed in Session 1).

TRANSITIONING TO THE FAMILY SESSION

Discuss the family session with the youth prior to inviting parents into the session. Provide the rationale for including family sessions in this treatment, including how parents can help support the youth in meeting any goals and preventing relapse.

IDEAS FOR THE THERAPIST	
Younger Youth	**Older Youth**
• Use Handout 5.6 (Depression Pie). • Have the youth explain the Self-Triangle to the parents. • Use more visual aids (white board, handouts). • Involve parents in the teaching/ psychoeducation of depression, relapse, and CBT. • Consider using parents in the development of the timeline. • For core skills, consider asking the youth to teach the skill to the parent.	• May contract with the youth to work on log of thoughts/behaviors related to mood prior to next session and to think about self-beliefs and evidence. • Send home the depression, relapse, and CBT educational material for review. • Use application to the child's situation early on. For example, once the CBT model is presented, ask the teen how it can be applicable to his or her situation. If you can go further, see how he or she can use that knowledge (mood/thought connection) during the following week. • Consider having the youth work on goals/ targets for change for homework. • Identify with the youth, and later with family, targets for change at home.
In this session, assess if the youth would respond better to more behavioral approaches or more cognitive approaches.	

First, review what will be discussed in the parent session.

• Work collaboratively with the youth to set a workable agenda for the parent session.

• Determine what issues would be helpful to discuss further.

• Determine any issues that the youth does not want to discuss during the parent session.

Family Session: Psychoeducation

AGENDA

Collaborate with the family to set an agenda for the family session.

• Elicit the family's input on the handout (from the waiting area).

• Review the CBT model and relapse prevention.

• Review expectations for therapy.

• Elicit parents' issues of concern about their child.

- Begin to gather information on past factors associated with the youth's depression (particularly family factors) and their input on current residual symptoms and anticipated future obstacles (add these to the timeline). Elicit parent input on treatment goals for the program.

- Remember to prioritize the agenda items collaboratively.

THERAPIST TIP: Do not show the timeline to the parents without the youth's permission. It really isn't necessary to show the timeline to the parents, as it is a tool for working with the youth individually. Collaborate with the youth to add family skills to the timeline, as needed.

TEACH AND PRACTICE

Rapport Building and Assessing Residual Symptoms

Ask parents to summarize the youth's past functioning. Be sure to ask about symptoms in the residual phase of depression.

- Tell the parents that you do have some information about the youth from previous treatment (initial assessments or referral information), so they do not need to go through the entire history, but that you would like to get a summary of what the teen's depression and treatment have been like from their point of view.

- List any important past or current symptoms to be added on the timeline with the youth in a later session.

- Remember to ask about the youth's functioning at home, in school, and with friends.

- Get the parents' point of view.

"What is the youth still struggling with? What has improved? What hasn't seemed to get better? Is there anything that is still concerning to you? What symptoms would you look for to recognize that your teen is getting depressed again?"

The CBT Model for Relapse Prevention

Introduce the CBT model.

- Introduce Handout 5.1, Self-Triangle. Provide an example to demonstrate the connection of each part of the self-triangle, emphasizing the reciprocal influence of the self-triangle. Each part of the triangle affects the other parts.

- Show the family Handout 5.3, My Relapse Prevention and Wellness Program, with each skill and what it will help with, to reinforce this idea. Elicit parent feedback about skills.

Review Expectations for Therapy

Review schedule of treatment, confidentiality, and attendance using Handout 5.4, Expectations. In addition, make sure the family is aware of contact information and is provided with emergency numbers and procedures.

- Troubleshoot any barriers to attendance and/or compliance.
- Begin with a suggested schedule and discuss with the patient and family.
- Introduce the schedule as flexible.
- Discuss the importance of communication and feedback. Any feedback is helpful; emphasize that you will use this feedback to make changes accordingly.

Treatment Goals

Discuss the parents' treatment goals for their child. Handout 5.9, Goals for My Child, is optional.

SUMMARY AND HOMEWORK/PRACTICE

Summarize the family session.

- Assess the family's understanding of CBT and the relapse prevention model.
- Elicit feedback about the session.
- Have the family summarize the session.

Collaborate to develop a family homework/practice assignment. Homework ideas include:

- Contract for the family to review the psychoeducational materials in the upcoming week.
- Have the family list goals for this treatment and bring them back for discussion.

DID IT STICK? (REVIEW QUESTIONS FROM THE SESSION)

1. What are the three parts of the self? How do thoughts and behaviors influence mood?
2. Why is the timeline important?
3. What can you expect to get out of this program?
4. How will parents be involved?

CASE EXAMPLE: SESSION 1

Lily is a 12-year-old Caucasian female who presented with her first episode of MDD to the clinic. Lily is in seventh grade and lives with her mother, father, and twin sister. The school counselor became concerned after Lily came to her office reporting thoughts of hurting herself, and the school counselor contacted Lily's parents. At the initial intake appointment, Lily's mother reported she had not been consistently attending school for the past 4 weeks, had few close friends, and described being "picked on" by her classmates. Her twin sister is a high academic achiever and socially extroverted, and Lily frequently compares herself to her sister. Lily is a talented artist, but her drawings had more recently included morbid content. Lily reported she had not enjoyed drawing as much lately, and she had dropped out of choir because "it's not fun anymore." Her depressive symptoms at intake included sad mood and irritability, anhedonia, sleep disturbance (hypersomnia), fatigue, suicidal thoughts, and feelings of guilt/worthlessness.

In the acute phase of treatment (6 weeks), Lily saw a pediatrician and received treatment with fluoxetine (30 mg/day). She responded well to medication treatment, remitting at 5 weeks. At Week 6, in addition to continuing the medication treatment, she began to meet with a therapist to address relapse prevention. The therapist began RP-CBT with Lily and her family at that time. Although she had some improvements in school attendance and performance, an assessment of residual symptoms revealed continued sleep disturbance and anhedonia. Lily reported that she was still taking naps after school every day and had trouble falling asleep at night. Additionally, she was not spending as much time on her art and continued to decline friends' request to hang out, stating, "They don't really like me, and I don't like hanging out with them anyway." The therapist completed the timeline with Lily (see Figure 5.1) and discovered that she also continued to struggle with self-deprecating thoughts, negative comparisons to her sister, and difficulty making friends.

RP-CBT began with an introduction to the idea of a continuation-phase treatment, specifically how adding therapy after improvement in depressive symptoms can help prevent relapse. The therapist used examples from Lily's recent stressors to illustrate how RP-CBT might be helpful to her. The therapist collaboratively set

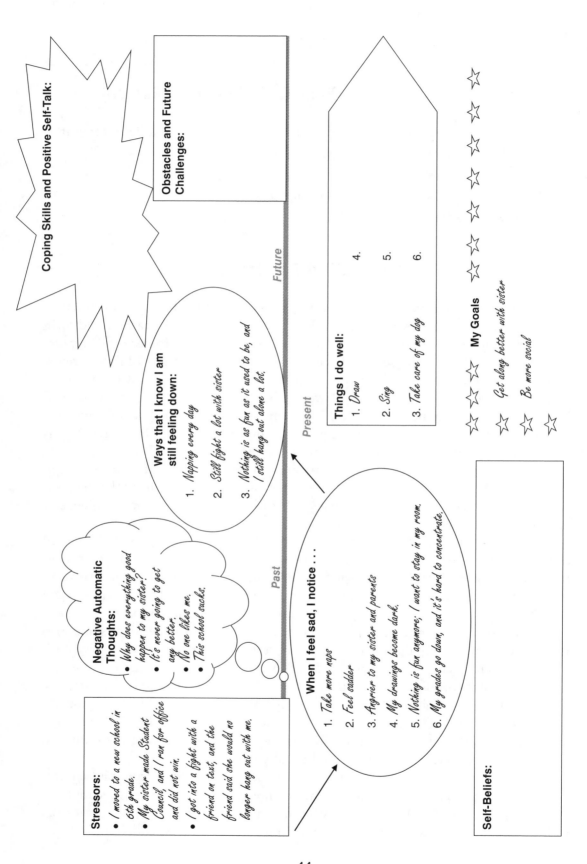

FIGURE 5.1. Lily's completed timeline during Session 1.

44

treatment goals with Lily. Lily wanted to work on being more social and not being as upset with her sister. These goals were tied to the timeline, specifically identified as "My Goals." The therapist and Lily moved through each section of the timeline together, thinking back to when Lily was the most depressed a few months ago, discussing stressors, common negative thoughts, and symptoms at that time. They then reviewed Lily's current difficulties, identifying these on the timeline as "Ways that I know that I am still feeling down."

The therapist asked Lily if she would be willing to track her mood and activities on Handout 5.2, Mood Monitor Log. She was also asked keep track of her sleep using a sleep diary. At the end of the session, Lily and her therapist completed a Make It Stick note to summarize the session and Lily's practice assignments.

The therapist met with Lily and her parents to review the CBT model (Handout 5.1, Self-Triangle). While reviewing Handout 5.8, The Basics of Depression, the therapist asked the parents for their perspectives on Lily's depressive symptoms before initially seeking treatment and currently. The therapist highlighted the parents' efforts to get Lily care when she needed it and emphasized the need for the parents to focus on reducing stress at home. As both Lily and her parents discussed concerns about the frequent napping, the therapist provided education about sleep and mood and gave them Handout A.6 with tips for improving sleep. Lily and her parents were provided with written materials to further educate them about relapse prevention and CBT.

Postcard reminders of the session content and the log activity (Figure 5.2) were sent before the next session.

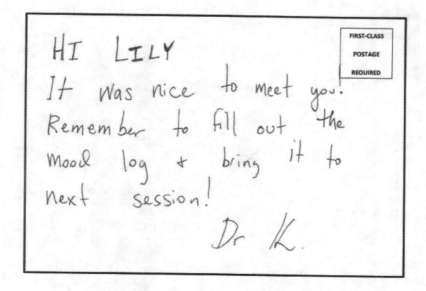

FIGURE 5.2. Postcard reminder after Session 1.

SELF-TRIANGLE

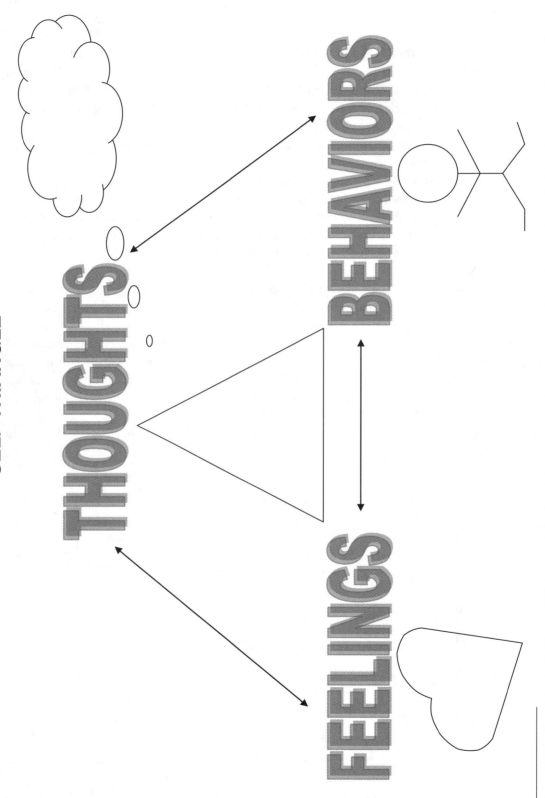

MOOD MONITOR LOG

	Situation	Feeling
Monday		
Tuesday		
Wednesday		
Thursday		
Friday		
Saturday		
Sunday		

MY RELAPSE PREVENTION AND WELLNESS PROGRAM

"The Basics"

- ☐ Introduction to the Program
- ☐ Behavioral Coping Skills
- ☐ Cognitive Restructuring and Automatic Thoughts
- ☐ Problem Solving
- ☐ Wellness
- ☐ Relapse Prevention and Wellness Plan

More Possibilities

- ☐ Adherence
- ☐ Anxiety
- ☐ Assertiveness
- ☐ Boredom
- ☐ Emotional Regulation
- ☐ Hopelessness
- ☐ Impulsivity
- ☐ Interpersonal Conflict
- ☐ Irritability
- ☐ Peer Victimization (Dealing with Bullies)
- ☐ Relaxation Training and Sleep Hygiene
- ☐ Social Skills
- ☐ Social Support
- ☐ Suicidality: Guidelines for Management

EXPECTATIONS

What should you expect from the therapist?

- Confidentiality unless you are in danger of harming yourself or others.
- Collaboration with you during therapy.
- Investment in keeping you well.
- Respect for your ideas and opinions.
- Open to feedback and willingness to adapt to your needs.

What does the therapist expect from you?

- Be on time and attend all sessions.
- Be prepared for each session.
- Be open and honest with the therapist.
- Invest in staying well.
- Be willing to give feedback.

What is the format for our therapy sessions?

- Provide parents with handout on today's topic while waiting.
- Set agenda.
- Review self-reports measures.
- Review previous session (Did It Stick?).
- Review practice from previous session and discuss any problems with the practice.
- Psychoeducation and skill teaching.
- Consider how the new skill fits on the timeline.
- Collaborate on practice assignment for the next week.
- Summarize the session (Make It Stick).

What are the stages of therapy?

- There will be 8 to 11 sessions (with more sessions available if needed).
- *Stage 1:* During the first 4 weeks of treatment, you and your family will come in weekly. Parents will be invited into sessions 1, 2, and 3 for the last 30 minutes.
- *Stage 2:* This stage consists of four sessions of treatment (once every other week for 8 weeks). Sessions can be individual or family, with a minimum of one family session.
- *Stage 3:* This stage consists of 12 weeks, with three optional booster sessions (can be individual or family depending on your needs), with a suggested schedule of meeting once per month.

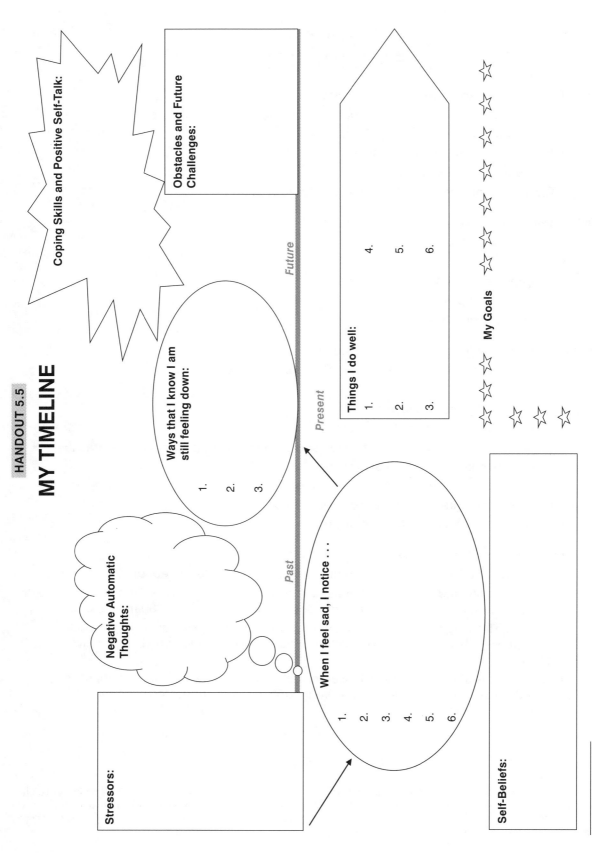

HANDOUT 5.5

MY TIMELINE

Coping Skills and Positive Self-Talk:

Obstacles and Future Challenges:

Negative Automatic Thoughts:

Ways that I know I am still feeling down:

1.
2.
3.

Stressors:

When I feel sad, I notice . . . .

1.
2.
3.
4.
5.
6.

Past

Present

Future

Things I do well:

1.   4.
2.   5.
3.   6.

My Goals

Self-Beliefs:

DEPRESSION PIE

How is your
depression
pie sliced?

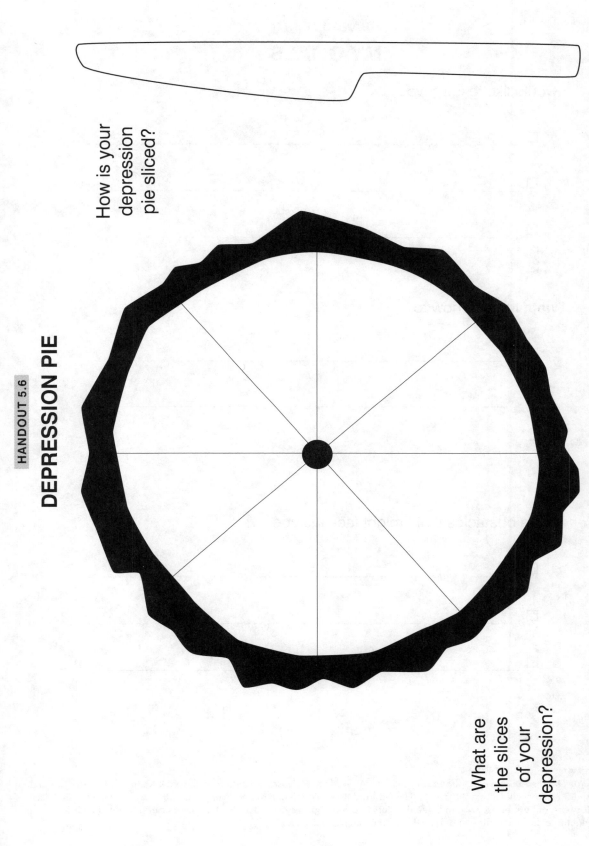

What are
the slices
of your
depression?

MY GOALS

I would like to improve . . .

☐ _____

☐ _____

☐ _____

I want to learn how to . . .

☐ _____

☐ _____

☐ _____

Future obstacles that I might face include . . .

☐ _____

☐ _____

☐ _____

THE BASICS OF DEPRESSION: PSYCHOEDUCATION FOR TEENS AND PARENTS

WHAT IS DEPRESSION?
Depression is an illness that affects your moods, thinking patterns, behavior, and motivations. Symptoms include:

- Sad, anxious, or bored mood
- Change in energy
- Slowing down of body or speech
- Change in sleeping patterns
- Change in socializing
- Hopelessness
- Suicidal ideation and/or behavior
- Irritability and/or anger
- Restlessness
- Loss of interest or pleasure
- Change in eating patterns
- Inability to concentrate or slowed thinking
- Guilt/worthlessness

MYTHS ABOUT DEPRESSION
- Depression will go away on its own.
- Everyone feels this way.
- The person with depression can control it and should be able to "pull him- or herself up by the boot straps" and feel better on his or her own.
- Depression is a sign of weakness.
- If a person talks about suicide, this means the person will not go on to attempt suicide.

HELPING YOURSELF
- Be hopeful—depression can be treated.
- Take medication as prescribed, even if beginning to feel better.
- Be direct in communicating.
- Be active in treatment.
- Keep a journal.
- Keep busy.

HELPING A LOVED ONE WITH DEPRESSION
- Changing expectations.
- Take care of yourself; go on with your life.
- Be direct in communicating.
- Provide feedback about positive changes you noticed.
- Always take suicide talk seriously—let us know.
- Make school aware of what is occurring—how teachers and staff can be supportive.
- Remember the illness is causing the person's changes—avoid taking angry comments personally.
- Look for gradual improvement.

TREATMENT OPTIONS
- Cognitive-behavioral therapy
- Family therapy
- Medications

Adapted from Poling and Brent (1997) and Kennard and Rush (1997) with permission from the authors.

GOALS FOR MY CHILD

I would like my child to improve . . .

☐ _____

☐ _____

☐ _____

I want my child to learn how to . . .

☐ _____

☐ _____

☐ _____

I plan to help my child by . . .

☐ _____

☐ _____

☐ _____

Future obstacles that my child may face . . .

☐ _____

☐ _____

☐ _____

CHAPTER 6

Session 2

Behavioral Coping Skills and Family Expressed Emotion

Use This Core Skill for . . .

- All youth to teach the core behavioral coping skills (behavioral activation) and identify targets for wellness and improved mood.
- All parents to discuss the importance of family communication and negative expressed emotion.

Session Objectives

- Introduce and practice activities to manage mood.
- Consider use of a wellness assessment, such as Handout 6.1, Wellness Log (see also Chapter 11), to ascertain the target areas of focus.
- Continue to explore past, present, and future symptoms using a timeline.
- Introduce self-beliefs and a positive self-schema.

Session Checklist

1. Provide the parents with a handout on today's topic while they wait.
2. Set the agenda; elicit the youth's agenda; evidence check (for or against self-belief).
3. Review self-reports (looking for possible residual symptoms).

4. Review the previous session (Did It Stick?, elicit feedback and summary, discuss results of homework/practice, discuss any adherence obstacles).

5. Teach behavioral coping skills and family expressed emotion.

6. Discuss and integrate results from any wellness assessment onto the timeline.

7. Perform homework/adherence check.

8. Elicit feedback and Make It Stick.

In this session, the first 45 minutes of treatment will be spent with the youth in an individual session, followed by a 45-minute conjoint session with the youth and parents.

INTRODUCTION

After going through items 1–4 of the Session Checklist, begin this part of the session. Assess the youth's understanding of the session model (i.e., that the session begins every time with setting an agenda, reviewing self-reports and the previous session, and homework). In addition, make sure the youth understands that sessions tend to be more helpful if the youth brings in ideas for the agenda, so that you can make the session more applicable to the youth's life and experience.

> *"When we're trying to learn to manage our mood, the first step is to learn to be aware of our moods. Later, it is important to look at patterns of our mood—how does it change during the day/week? Is there a relationship between our behavior and mood? Is there a relationship between our thoughts and mood?*
>
> *"There are two ways to manage mood: thinking and doing. Today we will focus on 'doing.' Mood changes are part of normal, everyday life. What is important to keep in mind is that managing mood is part of preventing relapse. If you find yourself being sad for a long period of time or over several days, we want you to be aware and take action to make sure that you don't get 'stuck' in the bad mood."*

THERAPIST TIP: Use the metaphor of a car being driven down the highway. There is a lot of traffic that day, and the other cars are going very fast, moving along. There will be bumps in the road and obstacles to increasing your speed or slowing down. It is easier to slow down, drive more skillfully, and be cautious through the bumps, rather than pulling off the road entirely, making it harder to get back into traffic (i.e., slowing down is a lapse versus pulling off the road, which is relapse).

RATIONALE

In this early part of the program, help the youth to identify mood states and to engage in simple activities to improve mood, when necessary. When one has been depressed, it sometimes becomes part of the way a person sees himself or herself. In addition, it becomes difficult to accurately gauge one's mood. For example, if a youth who has a history of depression feels sad about something, she may jump to the conclusion that she is depressed again. In all actuality, sadness and grief are normal and necessary emotions. When bad things happen, it is okay to feel these emotions. When a person has a history of depression, however, it is important to identify the intensity or degree of the sadness, grief, or irritability and to keep it from becoming too profound by doing something to bring up the mood (i.e., behavioral coping skill).

The goal is to have better control over mood and to be aware of changes in mood states so that one can intervene (by thinking and/or doing something to improve the mood state).

TEACH

Define "Mood"

- Mood is a term that relates to "feeling" or "emotion." Elicit the mood states of the youth that he or she is having the most problems with—for most youths, negative mood states can include sadness, anger, and anxiety or fear.

- Explain that moods are not all good or bad, but vary along a continuum. Identifying and measuring (or rating) these moods can be a helpful beginning tool in the management of mood.

- Can the youth give recent situations where he or she has felt very good? How about where he or she has felt very bad? What are the words attached to these mood states?

Monitoring Mood: What Is Your Temperature?

"One easy way to monitor your mood is to think of the range *of your mood as being like the numbers on a thermometer. When your number is low, like a 0 or 1, you feel calm or happy. When your number is high, like at a 10, your mood is sadder or angrier."*

You may choose to use Handout 6.2, Mood Thermometer. Have the youth fill in the thoughts and behaviors that go with each number on the thermometer on the handout. Note that the mood thermometer can also be used for emotions (e.g., irritability or anger) as well.

> **SUGGESTED HANDOUTS**
>
> ✓ Mood Thermometer (Handout 6.2)
> ✓ Feeling Faces (Handout 6.3)

Downward Spiral

Give an example of the downward spiral. Start with a stressor or an irritant. Show how thinking about this and dwelling on it brings the mood down. If one then stops activities, it brings mood down even more. This spiral can be compared to a snowball, rolling down a hill. As the snowball gains momentum, it gets bigger, which then makes it faster. This can be hard to control. It is easier to stop *before* it spirals out of control. Mood management skills can help with this (i.e., help to stop the snowball before it crashes at the bottom of the hill—relapse).

> **SUGGESTED HANDOUTS**
>
> ✓ Downward Spiral (Handout 6.4)
> ✓ Slippery Slope (Handout 6.5)

"Does this ever happen to you? Has it in the past? In this program you will learn ways to interrupt the downward spiral by changing your thinking or your behavior (using skills).

"Together we can find out what situations often lead to feeling bad, as well what situations or events lead to feeling good.

"Sometimes you find yourself in situations that can't be changed right away. We use different ways to cope with these situations. Also, the strategies that we will learn today will help you when you immediately need to shift your mood or if you are trying to prevent your mood from decreasing any more than it already has. These strategies can act as 'pick-me-ups.'"

Behavioral Coping Skills: Strategies for Mood Management

Introduce the idea of actions that bring mood up (behavioral activation/behavioral coping skills) and actions that bring mood down. Refer to Handout 6.6, Self-Triangle, and the idea of how this might help prevent relapse.

"We will <u>prevent relapse</u> through learning to manage mood—the first step is recognizing a downward spiral, and adjusting one's thoughts and/or behaviors to "catch" the mood before it spirals down.

"Can you think of things you do now that make you feel good? Try to find the links between doing and feeling. What about activities that lead to negative mood for you? Sometimes changing what you are doing can change your mood. Similarly, changing the way you think about a situation or view the situation can also change mood.

"One way to manage your mood is through activities that lift your mood—<u>behavioral</u> coping skills.

"Another way to manage mood is by monitoring your thoughts."

You may want to remind the youth of the triangle of mood and behavior and thoughts. The relationship between thoughts and mood is taught in the next session, but you may want to begin making this connection earlier.

The following is a list of behavioral coping skills—types of activities that counter depression and negative mood (Stark et al., 2007c).

1. Do something distracting and fun.

2. Do something relaxing and soothing.

3. Expend energy.

4. Do something social.

5. Do something that makes you feel successful: Mastery.

REQUIRED ACTIVITY

Using Handout 6.7, Behavioral Coping Skills, collaborate with the youth to make a list of these activities, and then work with the youth to make a plan for this week's practice. Consider using the Activity Scheduling handout for those youth who need more structure. Use examples to demonstrate the effect of behaviors on mood states. Consider using vignettes or in-session practice to demonstrate these concepts.

   1. Do something distracting and fun. List, with the youth, activities that are fun or that take his or her mind off of problems, negative mood. How often does he or she do these activities now? On the timeline, how often did he or she do these when depressed—is there a relationship between symptoms, mood, and activities over time?

2. Do something relaxing and soothing. Introduce the idea that people find different things relaxing. Make a list of relaxing and soothing activities with the youth. A checklist might help identify these activities. Suggest ways for the youth to do this, such as taking a bubble bath, doing breathing exercises or yoga, journaling, or listening to music.

3. Expend energy. Introduce the relationship between high-energy-expending activities and elevated mood. Adolescents who participate in regular exercise suffer lower rates of depression, and higher levels of general physical activity have also been related to lower rates of depression and feelings of hopelessness. Explore the relationship between high activity and mood over the past week, month, and on the timeline (e.g., did the youth ever go for a long run and feel "great" afterward?). To "expend energy" does not necessarily mean to engage in formal exercise. Suggest to the youth other ways to do this, such as dancing, walking the dog, active gaming, or taking the stairs.

4. Do something social. Social activities and social support are very important in elevating mood and in preventing relapse. Social support, or receiving support from others, and social altruism, or giving to others, are both important. Connecting with people gives one a sense of purpose and belonging. Introduce the concept of altruism as a part of well-being. Suggest to the youth ways to do this, such as helping a parent cook dinner or inviting friends over to play games.

5. Do something that makes you feel successful: Mastery. Feeling successful is associated with positive mood.

Consider the following questions: "What am I good at?" "What kind of person do I want to grow up to be?"

Look at the timeline, and explore the relationship between mastery and accomplishment and mood.

> **THERAPIST TIP:** Look out for perfectionism or negative thinking during this activity. Also, look for strengths and begin to build a positive self-schema.

> **SUGGESTED HANDOUTS**
>
> ✓ Behavioral Coping Skills (Handout 6.7)
>
> ✓ Activity Scheduling (Handout 6.8)
>
> ✓ Lift Your Mood (Handout 6.9)

PRACTICE IN SESSION

Have the youth use Handout 6.2, Mood Thermometer, to rate his or her mood for today. Have him or her rate yesterday's mood. What was the average reading when treatment began—in the acute phase? What is it now? What is different? Relate mood to current or past situations and thoughts if possible.

OPTIONAL ACTIVITY: **Thoughts, Mood, and Behavior**

- **Thoughts and mood:** Consider having the youth adopt a sample thought/or point of view and rate his or her mood. Then, change the thought and see how that might affect the mood rating.
- **Behavior and mood:** Sometimes just "acting" happy, or behaving as if one is happy, can actually result in a mood increase: Act happy/be happy.

OPTIONAL ACTIVITY: **Demonstrate the Behavior–Mood Link (Stark et al., 2007a) in Session**

"Can you remember the time you were the angriest or saddest?"

If the youth gives a time of grief, try to focus on sadness as different from a grief experience.

Have the youth engage in an activity that is pleasurable—jog in place/do jumping jacks/walk a flight of stairs—do this with the youth to help him or her feel less self-conscious.

Other suggestions include using a hula-hoop, tossing a ball, Nerf basketball free throws, or interactive computer games. Look for opportunities to make connections with the youth's interests.

Have the youth rate his or her mood before and after each experience or activity. What category would the activity fall into (fun, expend energy, mastery)? Some activities cross several categories.

THERAPIST TIP: The preceding activity is an example of helping the youth to apply the skill in the session. This treatment encourages this approach as much as possible, as this will help the youth to immediately apply use of the skill. Let the youth know the rationale for this: *"I like to try things in the session, to make a point and see if it changes how you feel."*

APPLY TO TIMELINE

"How would these strategies have helped you in the past?"

"How can they help you this week?"

"How can you use them in the future?"

The "apply" section is an opportunity to help the youth to identify *specifically* how the skill can be applied in his or her life.

"Can you think of ways to make your mood rating go up or down in your life? What about after the session or later this week?"

Try to start with an example that the youth gave in an earlier session. Is the youth aware of times in the past week when he or she felt badly? What are alternative ways to think about the situation; what are ways to change the behavior to get a change in mood?

OPTIONAL ACTIVITY: **Feedback on the Wellness Log**

If the youth is ready to work on wellness (see Figure 4.1 in Chapter 4), identify the areas of current strengths for the youth based on the Wellness Log (Handout 6.1). Validate that the youth has current strategies that are important for extending wellness. Discuss how these strategies developed, how he or she came to use them, and so on. Add these strengths to the timeline.

Look at areas where there is room for change. Does the youth see a connection between these wellness behaviors and extending the length of time that he or she is free from depression? Does he or she see a connection between higher wellness behaviors and lower stress/depression?

Is he or she interested in working on these behaviors? If so, which ones can be targeted this week? Which ones would he or she like to target in the future? Begin to introduce wellness and the rationale for wellness strategies in this treatment.

HOMEWORK/PRACTICE

Collaborate with the youth to identify how he or she can use what was learned in this session over the next week. Be specific!

"How might you practice behavioral coping skills at home this week?"

Brainstorm ways to overcome any barriers or obstacles to completing the homework. Remember to use a creative method of homework reminders, such as a between-session postcard, email, text message, or phone call!

"What is the likelihood that you will follow through on what is agreed upon for homework—how can we increase the percentage of likelihood of follow-through?"

Suggestions include:

1. Contract to have the youth keep a log of activities and a mood chart.
2. Contract with the youth to try two new behavioral coping skills this week. Consider sending the youth home with a journal to "catch" thoughts and

behaviors associated with negative mood. Look for high points in the week (Can the youth remember behaviors/thoughts around this point?).

3. If wellness concepts have been introduced, contract with youth to add new wellness strategies during the coming week.

MAKE IT STICK

Have the youth share what he or she learned in the session, and list these on a Make It Stick Post-it note. You can add any additional points to this list. The youth may also give feedback about what was the most helpful from the session. Share what you learned about the youth during this session (i.e., reinforce the youth's strengths).

In addition, you can create a postcard to send the youth during the week with the main points from the session. This should help the youth remember to practice what was learned in-session.

Suggested items for the Make It Stick include:

- Specific behavioral coping skills to use during the week. Have the youth list some that he or she is already good at (thus adding to positive self-schema), and have the youth list other areas where he or she may need to add some.

- Apply the skill to a specific, personal example.

IDEAS FOR THE THERAPIST	
Younger youth	**Older youth**
• Use vignettes. • Concrete example of behavioral activation. • Handout 6.9, Lift Your Mood. • Handout 6.3, Feeling Faces.	• Use real-life examples. • Consider finding a movie clip from a youth film to demonstrate behavioral coping.
More behavioral	**More cognitive**
• Consider rating mood in session, then add a pleasant activity—play games (tic-tac-toe toss across, horseshoes, Nerf basketball, hula hoop), then rate mood . . . • Use Handout 6.9, Lift Your Mood, to discuss: What brings your mood up? Things I can count on. What brings your mood down?	• Begin to introduce automatic thoughts or problem solving. • Introduce concept of thought check.

TRANSITIONING TO THE FAMILY SESSION

Discuss the family session with the youth prior to inviting parents into the session. First, review what will be discussed in the parent session.

- Work collaboratively with the youth to set a workable agenda for the parent session.

- Determine what issues would be helpful to discuss further.

- Determine any issues that the youth does not want to discuss during the parent session.

- Explain the concept of expressed emotion and how this relates to relapse. You will want to get the youth's "buy-in" and collaborate with the youth on how this concept may relate to his or her family and be helpful in the youth's treatment.

- Have the youth think about how this new family skill might be applied to the timeline. Consider what the family can do to help support the youth in preventing relapse.

THERAPIST TIP: Collaborate with the youth to make the determination about how much intervention versus psychoeducation needs to be done with the family. For example, low-expressed-emotion (EE) families may just need information on how sarcasm and criticism affect mood. High-EE families will need more work on reducing expressed emotion and communicating more effectively at home. High-EE families are at a higher risk for relapse, so more family intervention may be needed for these families.

Family Session: Expressed Emotion

AGENDA

Collaborate with the family to set an agenda for the family session.

- Check in with the family to make sure the psychoeducational materials (e.g., Handout 6.10, The Basics of Depression) have been reviewed and answer any questions about this material.

- Elicit feedback on the program and the past week. Continue to gather information on past factors associated with the youth's depression (particularly family factors) and their input on current residual symptoms and anticipated future obstacles (add these to the timeline). Continue to get parent input on treatment goals for the program.

- Elicit any questions parents may have after reviewing the parent handout. An optional agenda item is to have the youth teach the behavioral coping skills to the parents.
- Remember to prioritize the agenda items collaboratively.

TEACH AND PRACTICE

Introduce Expressed Emotion

"The communication and emotional level in a home can be thought of as being on a thermostat. The 'temperature' needs to be set at a level that is comfortable for all. This skill is particularly important because relapse in children and adolescents with depression occurs more frequently in families with high levels of negative emotion."

Use the metaphor of a good coach versus a bad coach.

"A good coach is supportive of the player, even when mistakes are made. Good behavior is praised, and bad behavior is corrected but with support and patience."

- Tie the idea of coaching style to parenting style. It is common in families in which there are members with depression to have negative emotion: sarcasm, high levels of criticism, and low levels of positive reinforcement/praise.
- Show Handout 6.11, Problem Communication Behaviors.

  "Which ones are true for your family?"

- Take time to normalize these situations. Most families interrupt or blame at times. Particularly in depressed families, people tend to feel overly accused. Use the metaphor of doing laundry:

  "I don't know about your family, but in my family we have a lot of dirty laundry. If one person were responsible for all of this dirty laundry, it would be overwhelming! But when each family member takes responsibility for his or her own stuff, no one has to deal with the whole mess. In families, every person has his role in conflict and communication. If everyone will take responsibility for their part in conflict, then it is a shared responsibility for the family to work on as a team." (K. Poling, personal communication, 2005)

- Contract with the family to begin to identify times when this occurs in their home. Consider reviewing Handout 6.11, Problem Communication Behaviors, with the family, discussing any examples that resonate with them.

  "Is it okay with you if I point this out when I see it occurring in the session?"

SUGGESTED HANDOUTS

✓ The Basics of Depression (Handout 6.10)

✓ Problem Communication Behaviors (Handout 6.11)

- Additionally, you may want to collaborate with the family on how much emphasis needs to be put on expressed emotion with this youth and family. If the family feels that high EE is an issue in their home, spend more time with interventions for this (see Optional Activities, below).

OPTIONAL ACTIVITIES

If the family has communicated that high EE is an issue for them, several interventions might be helpful.

1. Role-play both positive and negative communication with the family. After this, have family members point out the "right" and "wrong" aspects in the scenarios.

2. Help to dissect a recent conflict in the home, helping the family members to identify the roles played. Also, you can assist the family in recognizing any escalation points or "points of no return." Collaborate with the family to identify boiling points and come up with strategies to lower the family temperature at these points.

3. Have each family member discuss what he or she finds helpful about other family members' communication styles and what each would like to see more of (e.g., "I like it when you compliment me on my schoolwork, and I would like for you to comment about my artwork more."

4. You can invite families to bring disagreements or arguments from the home to your attention. These can be addressed in later sessions.

5. Introduce the idea of family behavioral coping activities. Collaborate with the family to plan an activity with a low risk of negative EE to increase the amount of positive interactions in the family.

SUMMARY AND HOMEWORK/PRACTICE

Summarize the family session.

- Assess the family's understanding of expressed emotion.
- Elicit feedback about the session.
    "How is this relevant to your family's situation?"
    "How can I, as the therapist, be helpful?"
- Have the family summarize the session.

Collaborate to develop a family homework assignment. Homework ideas include:

- The negotiation of an "escape plan." Have the family agree that when emotions get high, they will use the listening and communication strategies discussed in the session. Have the family report back on how these strategies worked for them.
- Have the family plan an activity to do in the upcoming week. This activity should have a low risk of conflict. Contract with the family to do this activity and report back on how it went.

DID IT STICK? (REVIEW QUESTIONS FROM THE SESSION)

1. What are behavioral coping skills—which types work for you?
2. Why should we monitor mood?
3. Why is it important in relapse prevention?

CASE EXAMPLE: SESSION 2

In the second session, Lily brings in her completed Mood Monitor Log and sleep diary. After setting the session agenda, Lily and the therapist review the practice assignments. In reviewing the Mood Monitor Log, it became clear that Lily's lower mood ratings were associated with conflict at home. In addition, the sleep diary indicated problematic sleep habits, including napping during the day and using her cell phone in bed to use social media. Lily reported continued improvement in mood, with less sadness, but also described continued irritability, in particular with her sister. She rated her average mood as a "5" on a 1–10 scale, with 10 being the worst mood.

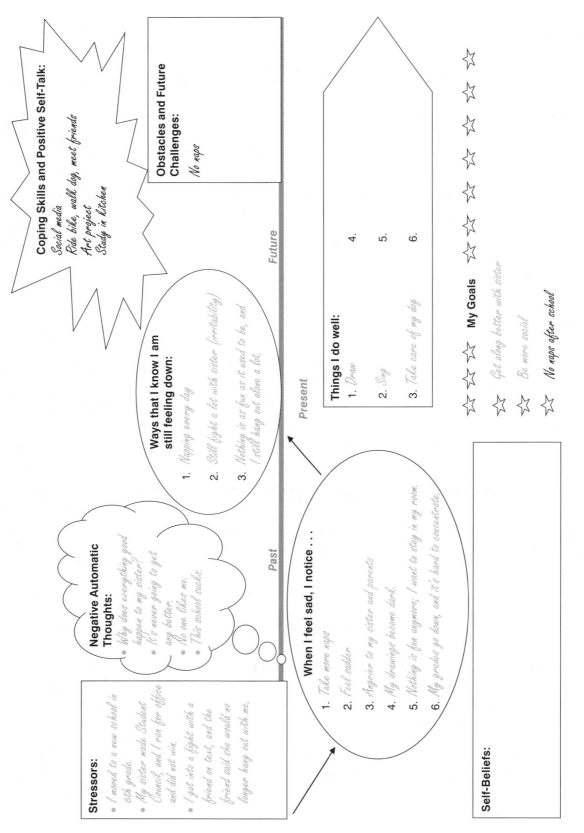

Stressors:
- I moved to a new school in 6th grade.
- My sister made Student Council, and I ran for office and did not win.
- I got into a fight with a friend on text, and the friend said she would no longer hang out with me.

Negative Automatic Thoughts:
- Why does everything good happen to my sister?
- It's never going to get any better.
- No one likes me.
- This school sucks.

Coping Skills and Positive Self-Talk:
Social media
Ride bike, walk dog, meet friends
Art project
Study in kitchen

Obstacles and Future Challenges:
No naps

Ways that I know I am still feeling down:
1. Napping every day.
2. Still fight a lot with sister (irritability).
3. Nothing is as fun as it used to be, and I still hang out alone a lot.

When I feel sad, I notice . . . .
1. Take more naps
2. Feel sadder
3. Angrier to my sister and parents
4. My drawings become dark.
5. Nothing is fun anymore; I want to stay in my room.
6. My grades go down, and it's hard to concentrate.

Things I do well:
1. Draw
2. Sing
3. Take care of my dog
4.
5.
6.

My Goals
☆ Get along better with sister
☆ Be more social
☆ No naps after school

Self-Beliefs:

Past   Present   Future

FIGURE 6.1. Lily's completed timeline during Session 2.

68

The therapist introduced the behavioral coping strategies as a way to reduce irritability and improve mood. The therapist commented that this set of skills could be particularly helpful given Lily's reported irritability and tied this idea to Lily's agenda item of getting along better with her parents and sister. Lily and the therapist noted that irritability had been listed as a residual symptom on her timeline (see Figure 6.1).

The therapist and Lily reviewed the five categories of behavioral activation skills, and Lily was able to identify several activities to fit within each of these categories:

- Distracting and fun: being on social media, watching TV series and movies.
- Relaxing and soothing: hot bath, reading a book.
- Expending energy: riding bike, taking dog for a walk.
- Social: texting a friend, going to mall with a friend.
- Mastery: art project.

The therapist and Lily planned how these activities could be used over the coming week to improve mood. In addition, they planned how she could use these strategies in response to irritability or conflict at home. They developed a specific homework/practice plan for the following week.

Lily and the therapist ended the session by planning for the family session. Lily stated that she thinks her parents still don't understand her depression. The therapist helped her identify ways that her parents could be more supportive. They agreed to this in the family session.

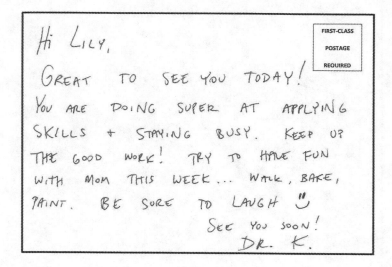

FIGURE 6.2. Postcard reminder after Session 2.

In the family session, the therapist collaboratively set the agenda, which included further psychoeducation about depression. Lily introduced behavioral coping skills to her parents and how they are relevant to her treatment and continued prevention of relapse.

The therapist highlighted the connection between problem communication behaviors and negative emotion and the risk for relapse. In the family session, the therapist worked with the parents and Lily to collaboratively determine ways to provide support to Lily. They discussed parents' expectations for Lily at home, which included wanting Lily to spend more time with the family, wanting her to stop taking so many naps, and requiring her to have planned study time daily at the kitchen table. The therapist and Lily worked with the family to call a truce on questions about schoolwork and grades and planned a few specific family behavioral coping activities for the week, including a family bike ride, game night, and breakfast at Grandma's on Sunday.

The therapist met with Lily's parents briefly at each visit to obtain input about her progress and to answer questions about the skills handouts provided to the parents at each session. A postcard reminder of the session content, which included a review of applying skills (see Figure 6.2), was sent before the next session.

WELLNESS LOG

Day	Self-Care	Self-Acceptance	Social	Success	Self-Goals	Spiritual	Soothing
	Sleep—What time I went to bed **Exercise**—Time I spent in activity **Food**—Things I eat	Positive statements that I say to myself	What I did for fun	Things that I was good at	My short-term and long-term goals	Times I spent in reflection or doing something for others	What I did to relax

MOOD THERMOMETER

Actions and Thoughts

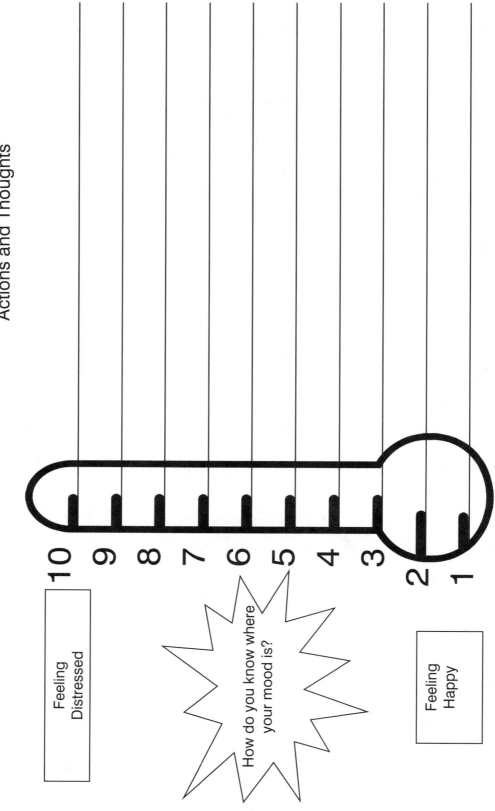

Feeling Distressed

How do you know where your mood is?

Feeling Happy

10 9 8 7 6 5 4 3 2 1

FEELING FACES

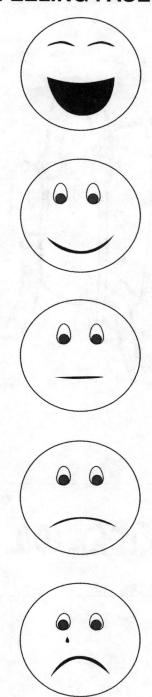

DOWNWARD SPIRAL

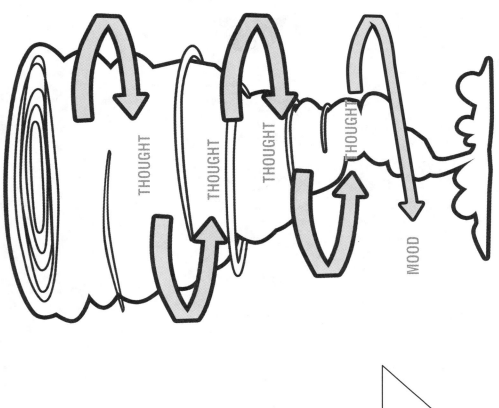

SLIPPERY SLOPE

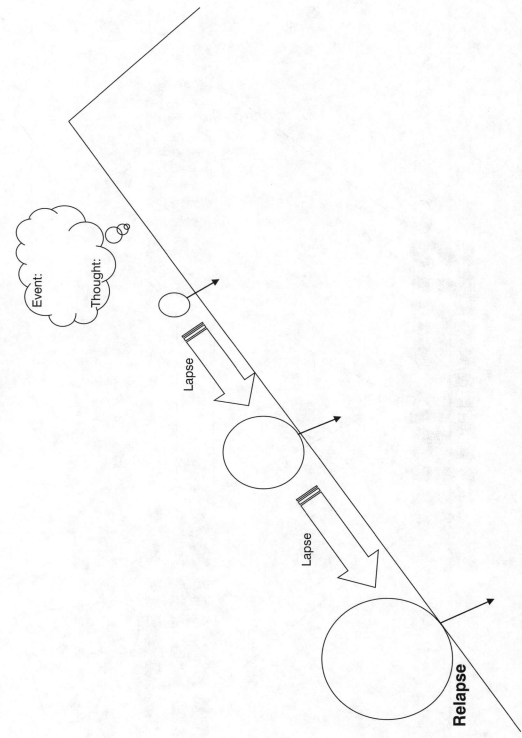

Event:

Thought:

Lapse

Lapse

Relapse

SELF-TRIANGLE

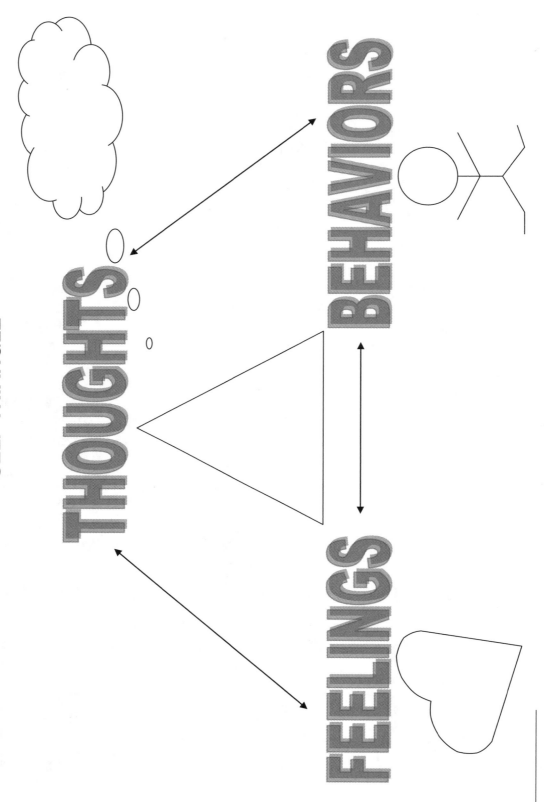

BEHAVIORAL COPING SKILLS

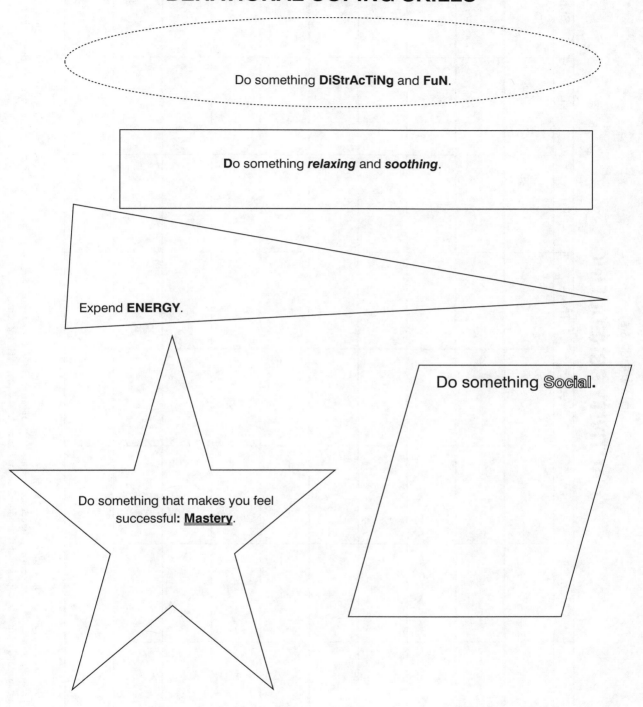

Do something **DiStRAcTiNg** and **FuN**.

Do something *relaxing* and *soothing*.

Expend **ENERGY**.

Do something Social.

Do something that makes you feel
successful: **Mastery**.

ACTIVITY SCHEDULING

Activity	Mon.	Tues.	Wed.	Thurs.	Fri.	Sat.	Sun.

LIFT YOUR MOOD

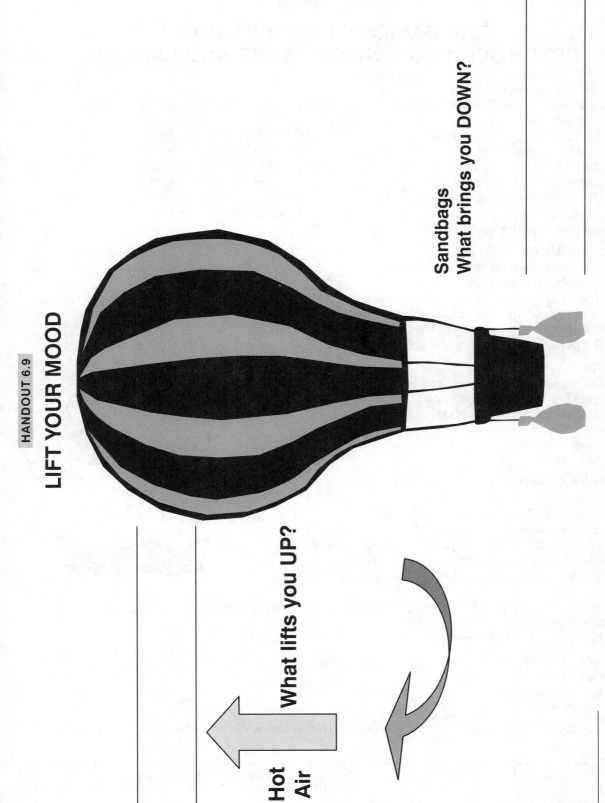

What lifts you UP?

Hot Air

Sandbags
What brings you DOWN?

THE BASICS OF DEPRESSION: PSYCHOEDUCATION FOR TEENS AND PARENTS

WHAT IS DEPRESSION?

Depression is an illness that affects your moods, thinking patterns, behavior, and motivations. Symptoms include:

- Sad, anxious, or bored mood
- Change in energy
- Slowing down of body or speech
- Change in sleeping patterns
- Change in socializing
- Hopelessness
- Suicidal ideation and/or behavior
- Irritability and/or anger
- Restlessness
- Loss of interest or pleasure
- Change in eating patterns
- Inability to concentrate or slowed thinking
- Guilt/worthlessness

MYTHS ABOUT DEPRESSION

- Depression will go away on its own.
- Everyone feels this way.
- The person with depression can control it and should be able to "pull him- or herself up by the boot straps" and feel better on his or her own.
- Depression is a sign of weakness.
- If a person talks about suicide, this means the person will not go on to attempt suicide.

HELPING YOURSELF

- Be hopeful—depression can be treated.
- Take medication as prescribed, even if beginning to feel better.
- Be direct in communicating.
- Be active in treatment.
- Keep a journal.
- Keep busy.

HELPING A LOVED ONE WITH DEPRESSION

- Changing expectations.
- Take care of yourself; go on with your life.
- Be direct in communicating.
- Provide feedback about positive changes you noticed.
- Always take suicide talk seriously—let us know.
- Make school aware of how teachers and staff can be supportive.
- Remember the illness is causing the person's changes—avoid taking angry comments personally.
- Look for gradual improvement.

TREATMENT OPTIONS

- Cognitive-behavioral therapy
- Family therapy
- Medications

Adapted from Poling and Brent (1997) and Kennard and Rush (1997) with permission from the authors.

PROBLEM COMMUNICATION BEHAVIORS

Problem Communication Habits	Positive Alternatives
• Accusing, blaming	• Making "I" statements ("I feel _____ when _____ happens")
• Using sarcasm	• Making communication direct, using a neutral voice
• Put-downs, name calling, shaming	• Accepting responsibility; making "I" statements
• Interrupting	• Listening quietly
• Lecturing, preaching, moralizing	• Identifying the problem; being brief
• Criticizing	• Identifying the positive; collaborating on solutions
• Mind reading (telling others what they think and feel)	• Asking people what they think and feel
• Getting off topic	• Catching onself and returning to the problem
• Dwelling on the past	• Sticking to the present and future (suggesting change to correct past problems)
• Monopolizing the conversation	• Taking turns making brief statements
• Threatening	• Suggesting alternative solutions
• Clamming up; not responding	• Reflecting; validating, expressing both negative and positive feelings
• Using "the silent treatment"	• Negotiating a later time to talk when everyone has "cooled off"

Adapted from the Treatment for Adolescent Depression Study (TADS).

CHAPTER 7

Session 3

Cognitive Restructuring and Identifying Unhelpful Thoughts

Use This Core Skill for . . .

- All youth to teach the core skill of cognitive restructuring and identifying unhelpful thoughts.

Session Objectives

- Introduce unhelpful thoughts and tie them to self-beliefs.
- Help the youth to identify his or her own unhelpful thoughts and to come up with helpful thoughts.
- Introduce the idea of self-beliefs (i.e., core beliefs) to the youth. Begin to conceptualize the youth's core belief.
- Describe the youth's attributional style for positive and negative events.
- Continue to identify unhelpful self-statements to target.

Session Checklist

1. Provide the parents with a handout on today's topic while they wait.
2. Set the agenda; elicit the youth's agenda; evidence check (for or against self-belief).
3. Review self-reports (looking for possible residual symptoms).
4. Review the previous session (Did It Stick?, elicit feedback and summary, discuss results of homework/practice, discuss any adherence obstacles).
5. Teach cognitive restructuring and unhelpful thoughts and self-beliefs.

6. Perform homework/adherence check.

7. Elicit feedback and Make It Stick.

In this session, the first 45 minutes of treatment will be spent with the youth in an individual session, followed by a 45-minute conjoint session with the youth and parents.

INTRODUCTION

After going through items 1–4 of the Session Checklist, begin this part of the session:

"It is easy to notice your feelings because that is probably what you are most aware of. It is key to recognize that there is a thought behind this feeling. For example, if you get a lower-than-normal grade back on a test, you may think, 'I am stupid. I will never pass.' Then this makes you feel bad about yourself, and this could make you feel like it is not worth trying anymore. The thought affects the feeling. Or, if you are at school and someone walks by and doesn't say 'hi' to you, you may think 'She doesn't like me.' But what if she is running late for class, or she didn't see you? The thought affects how you feel about yourself, but this thought may or may not be accurate."

RATIONALE

This skill will be needed by all youth who have dealt with depression. Actually, this skill would be useful for anyone who has ever had problems with "negative or unhelpful thinking" or has experienced cognitive distortions. Recognizing how one thinks and learning to identify the common errors in thinking will help to adjust these thoughts and to replace them with more accurate thoughts.

This skill helps to set the foundation for preventing relapse. In addition, this treatment focuses on self-beliefs, or core beliefs of the youth. By recognizing evidence for and against these core beliefs, the youth will hopefully be able to better manage his or her thinking and control his or her mood.

TEACH

Define Unhelpful Thoughts or Negative/Unhelpful Self-Talk

THERAPIST TIP: This section contains many suggestions for how to communicate this skill to youths. We suggest some possible language to use with youth to introduce this idea. Use anything needed to get the point across, but don't try to use it all. Use your best judgment of what will work best with your youth. If the youth "gets it," move on to the end of the section.

Thoughts and Mood

"When you are depressed, you feel bad, and in this treatment we focus on two factors that help maintain negative mood: thoughts and behaviors. In this session we focus on thinking patterns. Noticing the way you think is important to managing your mood and maintaining wellness. When you have thoughts such as, 'I did a great job with that,' do you see how that would make you feel better? When one is depressed, sometimes one learns to think negatively and practices this more. We need to evaluate your thinking patterns to see if some adjustment is needed to further improve your mood to prevent relapse.

"At times, there are some situations we can't change, such as parents' arguing. But you can change the way you think about it and how you cope with the situation (i.e., behavioral coping skills).

"Today we are going to talk about thoughts. Last week we discussed mood monitoring and ways to change your mood with behaviors. Today we are going to talk more about ways to change your mood by changing your thinking. Remember, your mood is affected by your thoughts, feelings, and behaviors. By working on changing your thoughts, we are also working on how to change your feelings, as thoughts can cause feelings."

The Role of Thoughts in Relapse Prevention

"You feel better now, but there may be some leftovers of the old thinking from when you were depressed. This leftover thinking may be keeping you from getting completely well. Today we are going to look at different ways that people think while they are depressed. Then, if it is okay with you, we are going to look at your thoughts and see if any of these ways of thinking have become your style of thinking. We are going to do a 'check' and see if any of these apply to you, then working on finding helpful ways of thinking, to prevent relapse in the future."

The language that follows may be helpful with youth who may need more examples to understand the connection between thought and mood.

"Even though you are feeling better, you may not realize that you are thinking that way because it becomes automatic. For example, when you first learned to ride your bike (or drive a car, play basketball, play

an instrument), you had to think about every move that you made. You focused on each detail of every sensation, such as movement, balance, and feeling. Then, after a while, you could do it without thinking—it became automatic. That is how thoughts are. When you were first depressed, you may have started to practice negative/unhelpful thinking. With time, that probably became the way that you thought most of the time. It may still be how you think—an automatic way of thinking—and this could cause you to feel down again. We need to relearn how to think—maybe give you practice thinking in a different, more realistic way. With practice, this will become your automatic way of thinking."

Changing Your Thoughts Is Possible

"Have you ever 'changed your mind' about something? How does the change happen? Did you question your old thought or get more information about something?"

- Introduce Handout 7.2, Risky Unhelpful Thoughts, and have the youth check those that apply to him or her.

> **SUGGESTED HANDOUTS**
>
> ✓ Downward Spiral (Handout 7.1)
> ✓ Risky Unhelpful Thoughts (Handout 7.2)

Strategies to Generate Helpful Thoughts: Thought Check

- **Check** to see if the thought is helpful. Check to see if the thought causes problems in mood (results in negative mood). *"When you experience a negative mood shift, that should signal for you to do a thought check."*

- **Challenge** the thought: Connect this to the triangle. *"How does this thought make you feel? What behavior does this thought lead to? Is this thought getting in the way of anything you want to do?"*

    ○ Contradictory evidence: *"What is the evidence for and against this unhelpful thought?"*

    ○ Alternatives: *"Is there another way to look at this (alternatives)? What would you say to a friend who has this thought?"*

    ○ Implications: *"If this thought is true, what is the worst that could happen? What is the best that can happen? What is most likely to happen?"*

    ○ Plan of action: *"When you have this thought, is there something you could do to change the situation or solve the problem?"*

- **Change** the unhelpful thought to a helpful thought.
  - Components of a helpful thought: realistic, makes you feel better, not extreme, not emotionally charged, not blaming.

> **THERAPIST TIP:** Beware of the "thinking trap"—"If I feel stupid, I must be stupid." Remind the youth that Handout 7.3, Thought Check, is appropriate in this case. The therapist might consider using Handout 7.4, My Self-Belief, to work on unhelpful beliefs. The youth might indicate a belief about him- or herself that is particularly unhelpful, such as "No one likes me." The therapist can indicate, using the circle as a pie chart, how much or what percent of all youth believes the particular belief to be true. For example, if it is 90% true, then the therapist can say, *"What would have to happen to get it to 80%?"* The therapist helps the child to find ways to reduce the belief—such as "I could go to the movie with a friend and I would believe it less." The therapist can illustrate this activity as a piece of the pie chart that reduces the 90% piece to an 80% piece. This activity can continue until the pie has several more "helpful" components to reduce the percent belief.

SUGGESTED HANDOUTS

✓ Thought Check (Handout 7.3)

✓ My Self-Belief (Handout 7.4)

Attributional Style (Ways of Explaining Things)

Attributional style can be twisted or skewed when one is depressed, and then people can get stuck in a pattern—for example, blaming yourself when things go wrong or not noticing or paying attention when things go well. Contract to explore with the youth his or her attributional style for both good things and bad things that happen. Research has shown that depressed adolescents have difficulty taking credit for positive events (i.e., depressed youth fail to make internal-stable-global attributions for positive events; Craighead & Curry, 1990). It is important for youths to "take credit" for good things that happen to them.

> *"We find that when good things happen to people who are depressed, they say it happened because of 'luck' or external situations (e.g., 'I made a good grade because the test was easy.'). It is important for us to watch for this. We need to make sure you give yourself credit for the things that you do well.*
>
> *"I would like to make a deal with you that during the treatment, I can point out when I notice that you are not taking credit for the good things that happen to you that you have had a part in. For example, if you study*

really hard and do well on a test, then tell me the test was 'easy,' I am going to remind you that you studied hard, and that is why you did well.

"Giving yourself credit for the things that you do well will help you to build positive self-beliefs, and these positive self-beliefs will protect you from relapse."

Self-Beliefs and Building a Positive Self-Schema

"We've been talking about how your view of yourself influences your thoughts and mood. We want to build a new idea of self that incorporates your strengths."

People have different ways of viewing themselves.

"For example, I am a therapist, a mother/father, a wife/husband, a daughter/son, and many other things."

In addition, people have ways of thinking about themselves.

"For example, I am smart, or funny, or serious, or likable."

These ways of thinking about yourself are called self-beliefs. These beliefs can be positive or negative (e.g., "I am smart" vs. "I am stupid"). Most people never really think about why they believe certain things about themselves, and that is too bad because these self-beliefs affect our thoughts, mood, and actions!

"For example, I think that I am stupid, so I don't raise my hand in class, even when I think I know the answer. What would happen if I believe that I am not stupid, or even believe that I am smart? How might my actions change? What would my mood and thoughts probably be like if I believe I am smart and try to answer questions in class?"

Discuss with the youth that a main goal of this treatment is to think about these self-beliefs and to try to understand any evidence that we have for these beliefs (good or bad) and against these beliefs (good or bad). Show the youth Handout 7.4, My Self-Belief, to better explain this concept.

"The ways that people view themselves can impact what they do. For example, if a person sees himself/herself as likable and fun to be around, he or she is likely to interact with other people. Self-beliefs (ideas or beliefs about myself that contribute to my mood, other thoughts, and behavior), both positive and negative self-beliefs, affect how we think, act, and feel. Let's

use this pie chart handout to think about 'how much' of you believes your most common self-beliefs.

"We just talked about a couple of beliefs you have about yourself. For example, 'I'm funny,' 'I'm stupid,' and 'No one likes me' [use actual examples from the youth, in his or her words]. What 'percent' of you believes each of these self-beliefs? Each of these beliefs is associated with different moods.

"When you say 'I'm funny,' your mood is much better. How can we increase the helpful self-beliefs and decrease the unhelpful self-beliefs? Both behaviors and helpful thoughts can change self-beliefs.

"If you want to decrease the 'stupid belief,' you can spend more time preparing for tests. In addition, you cannot minimize accomplishments (give yourself credit). Use the thought check method to address any frequent unhelpful thoughts about being stupid."

Common negative self beliefs include:

"I am unlovable."

"I am unworthy."

"I am not good enough. I don't measure up."

Use guided discovery to continue to uncover the youth's self-belief (e.g., "I noticed you said _____. Is that the way you see yourself?").

"Notice the good things you do. Which ones fit for you?"

Introduce the idea of monitoring helpful self-thoughts (or positive self-beliefs) and how these impact mood.

Apply the thought check model to the youth's negative self-beliefs, if possible.

SUGGESTED ACTIVITY: Flower Pot Metaphor

It may be helpful to guide the youth in understanding this concept by using the metaphor of a flower pot or gardening. If you fill the flower pot with rocks and sandy soil, then your plant will probably not be healthy and will have trouble growing to its full size. However, if you take time to tend the soil, add fertilizer, and pull out the weeds, you will find that the plant will thrive and reach its full potential!

Negative self-beliefs are like having sandy soil; no plant would grow well in this environment—think of the beach! There are not many plants on the shore!

Unhelpful thoughts are like the rocks in this sand, which inhibit the plant growth and mess up the roots.

Positive self-beliefs are the good soil, full of nutrients and life. Making positive attributions for events or "taking credit" for what you do is like adding fertilizer, and it makes your plant grow even better!

In this treatment, we would like to help weed the pot of the "bad stuff" (negative/unhelpful self-beliefs and unhelpful thoughts) and refill the pot with the good soil (positive/helpful self-beliefs) and fertilizer (positive attributes).

THERAPIST TIP: Continuously assess for the youth's self-beliefs and attributions for events. This is key in helping the youth to change how he or she thinks about the self!

PRACTICE IN SESSION

- Consider using Handout 7.2, Risky Unhelpful Thoughts, to help the youth practice finding the *unhelpful* thoughts.
- Role-play with the youth using yourself as an example. Give the youth a negative thought that you have had (e.g., "I was late to work this morning, so I am going to get fired."), and have him or her apply the thought check model. Try to connect negative thoughts with negative self-belief, if possible.

APPLY TO TIMELINE

"How would these strategies have helped you in the past?"

"How can they help you this week?"

"How can you use them in the future?"

If the youth has not already been able practice noticing unhelpful thoughts, help apply "thought check" to a specific thought that he or she has had over the past week. Go through the whole process with the youth's thought. Have the youth identify the thought behind the feeling and do a thought check.

- Past: *"What are some thoughts that you had when depressed? Or, if you can't remember, what do you think you were thinking back then, based on your symptoms? Knowing what you know now, could you talk back to these thoughts and change them?"*
- Present: *"Are any of these old thoughts still around?"*
- Future: *"Anticipate some situations for this week, and let's think of some positive self-statements that could be used in* that situation *(e.g., if third period at school is bad every single day, then anticipate some positive self-statements to use during this time)."*
- *"Make and keep a list of positive thoughts or self-statements that might work for you."*

HOMEWORK/PRACTICE

Collaborate with the youth to identify how he or she can use what was learned in this session over the next week. Be specific!
Suggestions include:

1. Thought record.
2. Make sure the Make It Stick includes common unhelpful thoughts for the youth to look out for during the week.
3. Use thought check cards: Have the youth make an index card with his or her common unhelpful thoughts and go through the thought check process with this card. Each unhelpful thought should have a helpful thought listed next to it. The youth can practice with these like flashcards.
4. Come up with some positive self-statements that could be used during the week. Have the youth anticipate situations in the upcoming week where these positive statements could be used. Incorporate positive self-statements into self-monitoring and the homework assignment.
5. Have the youth pay attention to the good things that happen in the upcoming week. Have the youth practice "taking credit" for these things.

MAKE IT STICK

Have the youth share what he or she learned in the session and list these items on a Make It Stick Post-it note. You can add any additional points to this list. The youth may also give feedback about what was the most helpful from the session. Share what you learned about the youth during this session (i.e., reinforce the youth's strengths).

In addition, you can create a postcard to send the youth during the week with the main points from the session. This should help the youth remember to practice what was learned in-session.

Suggested items for the Make It Stick include:

- Positive self-statements for the week ahead.
- Common unhelpful thoughts and helpful thoughts.
- Steps to thought check.
- Give self credit for events.
- Apply skill to a specific, personal example.

TRANSITIONING TO THE FAMILY SESSION

Discuss the family session with the youth prior to inviting parents into the session. First, review what will be discussed in the parent session.

- Work collaboratively with the youth to set a workable agenda for the parent session.

- Determine what issues would be helpful to discuss further.

- Determine any issues that the youth does not want to discuss during the parent session.

- Get the youth's "buy-in" and collaborate with the youth on how this concept may relate to his or her family and be helpful in the youth's treatment.

- Have the youth think about how this new family skill might be applied to the timeline. Consider what the family can do to help support the youth in preventing relapse.

IDEAS FOR THE THERAPIST	
Younger youth	**Older youth**
• Use vignettes. • Instead of common distortions, simplify into "red flag" words. • Which ones might he or she "catch" this week? • Ask permission to use Mom or Dad or a significant other to help the youth to catch the red flag words; can they "catch" them as a family? • Handout 6.9, Lift Your Mood.	• Use real-life examples. • Where are the unhelpful thoughts on this youth's timeline? • How can this skill be used to prevent relapse? • Have the youth consider how the self-belief gets in the way.
More behavioral	**More cognitive**
• State the thought and then rate the feeling in the session. • Have the youth teach the parent about unhelpful thoughts. • Use Handout 6.3, Feeling Faces. • Play Nerf football/basketball, having the youth describe thoughts after missing and making shots.	• Use Handout 7.2, Risky Unhelpful Thoughts; which ones are familiar? • What situations does the youth anticipate this week where he or she might catch the thought? • Thought journaling.

Family Session: Cognitive Restructuring

AGENDA

Collaborate with the family to set an agenda for the family session.

- Check in with the family on any previously assigned homework.
- Elicit feedback on the program and the past week. Continue to gather information on past factors associated with the youth's depression (particularly family factors) and their input on current residual symptoms and anticipated future obstacles (add these to the timeline). Continue to get parent input on treatment goals for the program.
- Elicit any questions parents may have after reviewing the parent handout. An optional agenda item is to have the youth teach the cognitive restructuring and unhelpful thoughts to the parents.
- Remember to prioritize the agenda items collaboratively.

TEACH AND PRACTICE

Introduce Cognitive Restructuring and Unhelpful Thoughts

- Remind parent and youth of the cognitive model of depression and bring out the triangle.

  "In this program, youth are taught to identify thoughts and attributions and challenge and change unhelpful thinking. This same process can be very helpful to parents."

- Introduce the idea that negative/unhelpful thoughts run in families.

  "Do you have any negative/unhelpful thoughts about yourself?"

- Identify negative attributions that the parent has regarding him- or herself, the world, or the future. Be alert to opportunities to teach developmental norms for youth. Many adolescents exhibit thinking that is self-focused. This is normal for this age group and is not necessarily pathological.
- Parents often have unhelpful thoughts regarding their depressed adolescent. These thoughts can increase parent–child conflict and solidify the negative automatic thoughts of the adolescent.
- Use Handout 7.2, Risky Unhelpful Thoughts, as a teaching tool to show examples of automatic thoughts. Have the family brainstorm any negative/unhelpful thoughts about their family or about each other, such as "Dad is never home" or "Mom is always on the phone" or "My brother is lazy." Have the family practice the thought check method, taught earlier in-session to the youth.

SUMMARY AND HOMEWORK/PRACTICE

Summarize the family session.

- Assess the family's understanding of cognitive restructuring and unhelpful thoughts.
- Elicit feedback about the session.

    "How is this relevant to your family's situation?"

    "How can I, as the therapist, be helpful?"

- Have the family summarize the session.

Collaborate to develop a family homework assignment. Homework ideas include the following:

- Contract with the family to have members point out to each other when they hear a negative or "unhealthy" attribution or statement. How can this be pointed out, without seeming critical? Have the family report back on some of these thoughts in a later session. For families with high EE, this may not be a good idea.

- Have each member of the family keep a mood monitor journal where thoughts are recorded. These do not have to be shared with each other but would serve as an exercise for individual reflection.

- As an experiment, have the family designate a "daily affirmation time." Practice making affirming statements about each member of the family. Then assess the result of this on the family environment and the mood of family members. Designate a time of day when family members regularly get together (such as dinnertime).

DID IT STICK? (REVIEW QUESTIONS FROM THE SESSION)

1. What are automatic unhelpful thoughts? What positive self-statements do you need to increase with practice?
2. Why should we "catch" them?
3. How are they important in relapse prevention?
4. Self-beliefs—What is my negative or positive self-belief? What can I do when I notice thoughts that contribute to my negative self-belief?

CASE EXAMPLE: SESSION 3

In Session 3, the therapist and Lily reviewed the behavioral coping practice that she did over the past week, noting that her mood did improve after she took the dog for a walk or worked on her art projects. She found it hard to do the activities on days that she was feeling sadder or was stressed about her school work. The therapist and Lily discussed scheduling one coping activity a day and explored how to include parents in helping her to stick to this schedule.

The therapist introduced unhelpful thoughts and their relationship to mood and behaviors and relapse prevention. Lily was able to identify several recurring unhelpful thoughts (e.g., "I'm stupid," "My parents love my sister more than they love me," and "I will never have friends."). Lily was able to understand the connection between these thoughts and negative mood. In addition, she could link the thoughts to her behavior and current situation (e.g., "I'm stupid" would lead to not even trying to study for a test; "My parents love my sister more, so I am not important and don't matter" would lead to her staying in her room and sleeping; "I will never have friends" would lead to avoiding talking to people at school).

The therapist introduced strategies to generate helpful thoughts, using the thought check skill. In the session, the therapist and Lily worked on the thought "I am stupid." This is a thought that Lily could tie to increased sadness and hopelessness. The therapist and Lily used the check, challenge, and change approach:

- *Check:* The thought was unhelpful due to its resulting negative mood, as well as a tendency to "give up" or not try in school.

- *Challenge:* Several strategies were used to challenge the thought. Contradictory evidence was identified, including that Lily was a straight A student prior to her onset of depression. In addition, she recently has been getting good grades in her English classes and has only one subject that is difficult for her. Lily used the alternative thoughts strategy to generate helpful thoughts, including "I am able to do better work," "I am good at many things," and "Lots of people struggle in math who are smart."

- *Change:* Lily wrote down the alternative thoughts above on a coping card. She set the goal of practicing saying these thoughts to herself whenever she struggles in math or feels down about school. In addition, she decided that she would spend more time after school on her homework. These alternative thoughts were added to the timeline (see Figure 7.1). Once she identified this pattern of thinking, Lily was able to plan ahead for when to use the thought check skill.

The therapist ended the session by planning for the family session with Lily and assigning a thought record for homework.

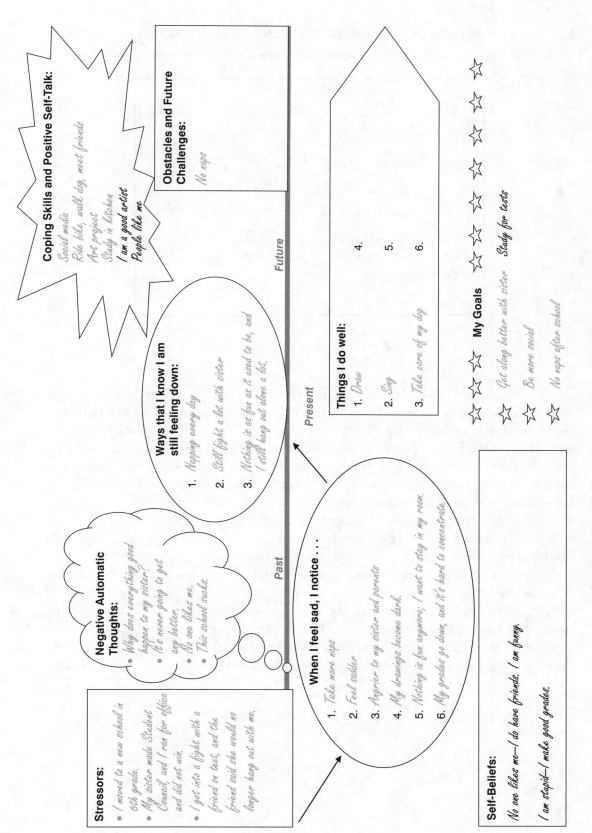

Stressors:
- I moved to a new school in 6th grade.
- My sister made Student Council, and I ran for office and did not win.
- I got into a fight with a friend or text, and the friend said she would no longer hang out with me.

Negative Automatic Thoughts:
- Why does everything good happen to my sister?
- It's never going to get any better.
- No one likes me.
- This school sucks.

Coping Skills and Positive Self-Talk:
Social media
Ride bike, walk dog, meet friends
Art project
Study in kitchen
I am a good artist
People like me

Obstacles and Future Challenges:
No naps

Ways that I know I am still feeling down:
1. Napping every day
2. Still fight a lot with sister
3. Nothing is as fun as it used to be, and I still hang out alone a lot.

When I feel sad, I notice . . .
1. Take more naps
2. Feel sadder
3. Angrier to my sister and parents
4. My drawings become dark.
5. Nothing is fun anymore; I want to stay in my room.
6. My grades go down, and it's hard to concentrate.

Past   Present   Future

Things I do well:
1. Draw   4.
2. Sing   5.
3. Take care of my dog   6.

My Goals
Get along better with sister   Study for tests
Be more social
No naps after school

Self-Beliefs:
No one likes me—I do have friends, I am funny.

I am stupid—I make good grades.

FIGURE 7.1. Lily's completed timeline during Session 3.

95

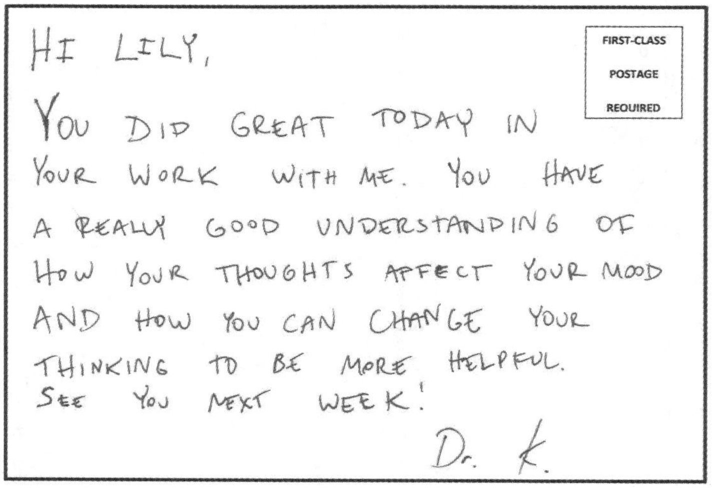

Hi Lily,

You did great today in your work with me. You have a really good understanding of how your thoughts affect your mood and how you can change your thinking to be more helpful. See you next week!

Dr. K.

FIRST-CLASS
POSTAGE
REQUIRED

FIGURE 7.2. Postcard reminder after Session 3.

The therapist asked, "What unhelpful thoughts might be useful to review with your parents?" They identified Lily's tendency to compare herself to her twin and her belief that her parents valued her sister more than they did her. In the family session, the therapist asked Lily to explain the connection between unhelpful thoughts and mood to her parents. She discussed her belief that they loved her sister more than her. Her parents and Lily used the thought check skill together to address Lily's unhelpful thoughts about her role in the family. The parents were able to point out how at times it seemed that Lily ignored the positive statements that they have made to her. In addition, the parents identified some unhelpful family beliefs, "Lily does not want to be around us," which resulted in the parents not planning family activities. The parents were more aware of Lily's feeling criticized, and they made a plan of action. They would try to be more aware of her unhelpful thinking and would provide more support. In addition, the family planned two family activities for the week, and Lily agreed to participate. The therapist sent a postcard over the next week (see Figure 7.2), which included a review of thought check and a reminder to practice using her helpful thoughts and to follow through with the family activities.

DOWNWARD SPIRAL

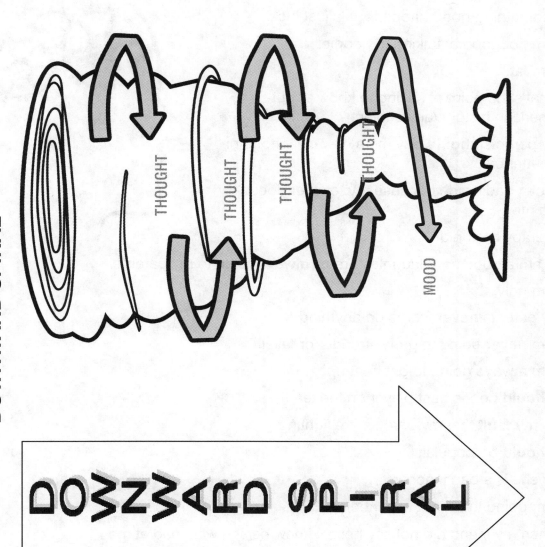

THOUGHT

THOUGHT

THOUGHT

THOUGHT

MOOD

DOWNWARD SPIRAL

RISKY UNHELPFUL THOUGHTS

☐ I am **never** going to have a boyfriend/girlfriend.

☐ If something good happens, it is just luck.

☐ I am not good at talking to people.

☐ I am fat.

☐ What's the point of having to know about American history (any subject)?

☐ My parents **should** buy me a new cell phone or a better car.

☐ I got a bad grade because my teacher doesn't like me.

☐ Therapy is stupid!

☐ If I am a good son/daughter, I must **always** listen to my parents.

☐ I am ugly.

☐ My parents **never** let me do anything.

☐ I am **never** going to grow stronger or taller.

☐ I am **always** going to get beat up.

☐ I **should** be the best player on the team.

☐ It's **my fault** that my parents are fighting.

☐ I **should** be popular.

☐ He/she is a bad teacher.

☐ I am going to fail out of school.

☐ When my friend did not say hello, I knew he/she was mad at me.

☐ I don't want to go to school (any activity).

☐ As a good friend, I **should** be supportive no matter what.

☐ If my team loses, it will be **my fault**.

Adapted from TADS manual.

THOUGHT CHECK

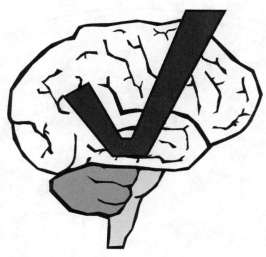

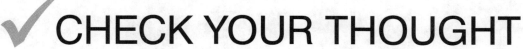

✓ CHECK YOUR THOUGHT

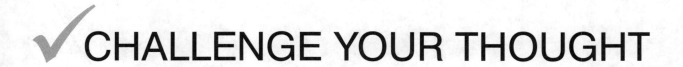

✓ CHALLENGE YOUR THOUGHT

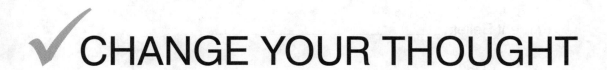

✓ CHANGE YOUR THOUGHT

MY SELF-BELIEF

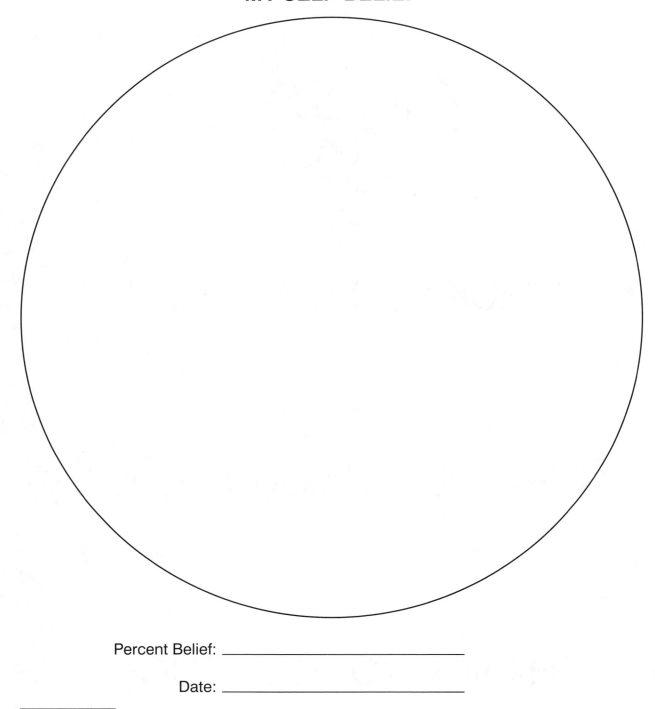

Percent Belief: _____

Date: _____

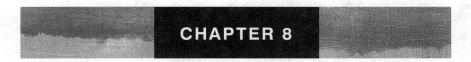

CHAPTER 8

Session 4

Problem Solving

Use This Core Skill for . . .

- All youth to help with problem solving.
- A youth who has difficulty in coming up with solutions to everyday problems.
- A youth who has trouble recognizing problems and thus solving them as such.
- A youth who presents a problem or dilemma during agenda setting.

Session Objectives

- Learn to define a problem and/or to identify common problems.
- Understand FLIP and how to use this approach when problem solving.
- Apply FLIP to a specific, personal problem.

Session Checklist

1. Provide the parents with a handout on today's topic while they wait.
2. Set the agenda; elicit the youth's agenda; evidence check (for or against self-belief).
3. Review self-reports (looking for possible residual symptoms).
4. Review the previous session (Did It Stick?, elicit feedback and summary, discuss results of homework/practice, discuss any adherence obstacles).
5. Teach problem solving.
6. How does this skill fit in on the timeline?

7. Perform homework/adherence check.

8. Elicit feedback and Make It Stick.

INTRODUCTION

After going through items 1–4 of the Session Checklist, begin this part of the session.

> *"Everyone faces problems in life, whether with family, friends, teachers, or co-workers. It is important to have a general way to solve these problems so that they don't lead you to feel discouraged, hopeless, or even depressed again.*
>
> *"You mentioned that you were struggling with _____ [give example of a problem on the agenda]. Today I wanted us to talk about problem solving and how this skill might help you solve this problem and future problems."*

Point out that in earlier sessions, the youth learned ways of coping with situations that cannot change (through use of behavioral coping skills and cognitive restructuring). Stress that this skill (problem solving) is useful when the situation can be changed.

RATIONALE

Problem solving is a useful skill in every aspect of life. The best way to deal with a lot of issues that upset you is to change them. This may sound easy, but it takes practice to brainstorm all options and pinpoint the best one for the situation. Refer to common problems that the youth has brought up, such as social and family conflict, academic problems, or problems with homework completion (see the Adherence Supplement in the Appendix for this problem as well). If the youth included a problem on the agenda, use this problem as an example.

TEACH

Define "Problem"

> *"What is a problem? Basically, a problem is a dilemma in which you have to make a choice about something or any situation that causes you to be anxious, worried, or stressed out. A problem can be a source of stress."*

Have the youth list some of his or her own problems from the past or present or anticipated problems in the future.

"Now that we both have a better understanding of what problems are, let's talk about solving them! It is important to have a general strategy for problem solving."

SUGGESTED HANDOUTS

✓ FLIP the Problem (Handout 8.1)

✓ FLIP the Problem (Example) (Handout 8.2)

Problem Solving: FLIP

"When you encounter a problem, FLIP the problem to look at all sides."

F: Figure out what the problem is and what you want to happen.

L: List all possible solutions.

I: Identify the best solution.

P: Plan what to do next.

F: Figure out what the problem is and what you want to happen.

"Sometimes when people are overwhelmed, it can seem like everything in life is part of the problem. This often leads to more stress! In order to solve the problem, you need to figure out exactly what the problem is."

L: List all possible solutions.

"Even adults often overlook this step in problem solving. Most problems have many possible solutions. The trick is to brainstorm all of these possibilities before choosing one. It is really important to focus on all possibilities without judging the solutions at this point. No potential solution is bad."

I: Identify the best solution.

"Once you have listed all possible options, you can fill in the positive consequences ('pluses') and negative consequences ('minuses') of each one. After looking at the positives and negatives of each option, it often is easy to choose a solution—the one with the most 'pluses'! If it is not obvious which solution is the best, then continue to brainstorm any 'pluses' or 'minuses' that you might have left off the list."

P: Plan what to do next.

"After choosing a solution, it is important to plan how to carry out this solution. Once you have acted on this solution, evaluate how it worked and how you feel about the problem now. If the problem still causes you stress, FLIP the problem again and come up with some new ideas."

PRACTICE IN SESSION

Have the youth help you to apply FLIP to either (1) his or her own problem or (2) a problem of someone else. There are some youth who have a hard time verbalizing one of their own problems. In this event, it is fine to use a vignette or sample problem in order to teach the steps in the skill.

> **THERAPIST TIP:** List some solutions that are extreme or unlikely to emphasize that, while brainstorming, you are just listing, not evaluating, the solutions. That comes in the next step, Identify.

APPLY TO TIMELINE

"How would these strategies have helped you in the past?"

"How can they help you this week?"

"How can you use them in the future?"

Have the youth anticipate a problem that is coming up in the week ahead. Have the youth FLIP the problem to see all sides. Help the youth to brainstorm specific details about the solution to this problem and to anticipate any "bumps in the road" that may come up while applying FLIP.

HOMEWORK/PRACTICE

Collaborate with the youth to identify how he or she can use what was learned in this session over the next week. Be specific!

Suggestions include:

1. Anticipate the problem in the week ahead, such as having trouble at school or home. Apply FLIP and report back on how it worked.

2. Come up with some positive/helpful self-statements that could be used during the week. Have the youth anticipate situations in the upcoming week when

these positive statements could be used. Incorporate positive self-statements into self-monitoring and homework assignments.

3. Have the youth pay attention to the good things that happen in the upcoming week. Have the youth practice "taking credit" for these things.

Contract with the youth to complete a Wellness Log over the following week if the youth is completing wellness at this point (see Figure 4.1 in Chapter 4).

SUGGESTED HANDOUT

✓ Wellness Log (Handout 8.3)

MAKE IT STICK

Have the youth share what he or she learned in the session and list these items on a Make It Stick Post-it note. The therapist can add any additional points to this list. The youth may also give feedback about what was most helpful from the session. Share what you learned about the youth during this session (i.e., reinforce the youth's strengths).

In addition, the therapist can create a postcard to send the youth during the week, with the main points from the session. This should help the youth remember to practice what was learned in-session.

Suggested items for the Make It Stick include:

- Definition of "problem"
- FLIP method steps
- Application of skill to a specific, personal example

IDEAS FOR THE THERAPIST	
Younger youth	**Older youth**
• Have the youth apply FLIP to an example problem. • Bring in the family and have the youth teach the skill to his or her parents.	• Have the youth apply FLIP to some of his or her own common problems.
More behavioral	**More cognitive**
• Role-play in-session. Contract to do FLIP this week (may include parents in the contract).	• How might this skill fit on the timeline—how might it have been used on a past problem? What about a current problem or future problem?

Family Check-In

DID IT STICK? (REVIEW QUESTIONS FROM THE SESSION)

1. What is problem solving, and why is it important?
2. What are some common problems that people encounter?
3. Describe how to FLIP a problem to see all sides.

CASE EXAMPLE: SESSION 4

In Session 4, the therapist and Lily reviewed the thought record that Lily completed over the past week. She was able to identify unhelpful thoughts related to school and at home. Of note, Lily used the check, challenge, and change strategies in order to change her unhelpful thoughts to more helpful/positive ones. Lily also noted that she actually enjoyed the family activities, and she expressed interest in planning more activities in the upcoming week. Lily reported an increase in mood rating (from 5 to 3) when she used cognitive restructuring at home and school.

The therapist and Lily set the agenda for the session, and the therapist introduced problem solving. On the agenda, Lily reported that she wanted to address her difficulty in finding fun things to do with friends. She explained that prior to being depressed, she was very socially active. However, lately she has been avoiding hanging out with friends, preferring to stay home and watch TV in her room. To tie the new skill to Lily's agenda item, the therapist asked, "How would it be for you if we used the problem you put on the agenda today to practice FLIP, a strategy for making changes in your life?" Lily agreed, and the therapist and Lily collaboratively completed the FLIP handout as follows:

F: First, Lily was able to figure out that the problem was that she was spending too much time alone. In addition, she could state that she wanted to be with friends more often and have fun.

L: Lily was able to list several possible solutions to address this problem. She listed activities that she used to like to do for fun as well as several friends she could approach easily. At first, she wrote down some activities that she said she no longer liked to do. The therapist reminded her that she could evaluate the options at a later step, but for now, she should focus on generating all ideas without judgment. Having just learned the cognitive restructuring skill, Lily was asked by the therapist to consider what thoughts might be helpful in this process. Those thoughts were put on the list as well—including "I can do this; I have had many friends before and I can again."

I: Lily was able to go through and evaluate each solution, using a plus sign for solutions that might work and a minus sign for those that would be less optimal or have a potential negative consequence (such as re-connecting with a friend that brings her mood down).

P: She was able to "pick and plan" as the final step. She decided to try to invite a friend to meet her at the movies to see a new film based on their favorite book. Lily role-played with the therapist how she would ask the friend to join her. They also discussed what support she might need from her parents, such as getting a ride to the movies. She also identified some helpful thoughts, such as, "It will be fun to see her," and "I used to love going to the movies with her," to aid her in successfully using the plan.

The parents were included at the end of the session to review the skill and Lily's plan to work on increasing her social activities. Lily was able to explain the FLIP method for problem solving to her parents. In addition, the problem-solving skill was discussed as one that could be used by the family. They discussed using the FLIP skill at home as a tool to reduce conflict and negotiate solutions. Lily and her parents discussed a fight that she and her sister had about how much time Lily's sister spends getting ready in their shared bathroom in the mornings. The family agreed to use the FLIP strategy as a family to address this issue and devise a plan.

Homework was assigned to practice using FLIP in the next week both at school and at home.

FLIP THE PROBLEM

F

> ***FIGURE OUT*** what the problem is and what you want to happen

L

> ***LIST*** all possible solutions

I

> ***IDENTIFY*** the best solution

P

> ***PLAN*** when and where to use this strategy

FLIP THE PROBLEM (EXAMPLE)

F

FIGURE OUT what the problem is and what you want to happen

Made a low grade on the test

- I would like to make a higher grade next time.

L

LIST all possible solutions

- Study with a friend
- Ask the teacher for help
- Make a study schedule
- Get a tutor
- Change classrooms or teachers
- Read the chapter several times

I

IDENTIFY the best solution

Make a study schedule

P

PLAN when and where to use this strategy

1. Create a weekly schedule and block off time to study
2. Begin the schedule a week before the test
3. Make flashcards and review during study time
4. Studying can be done on the kitchen table

WELLNESS LOG

Day	Self-Care	Self-Acceptance	Social	Success	Self-Goals	Spiritual	Soothing
	Sleep—What time I went to bed **Exercise**—Time I spent in activity **Food**—Things I eat	Positive statements that I say to myself	What I did for fun	Things that I was good at	My short-term and long-term goals	Times I spent in reflection or doing something for others	What I did to relax

CHAPTER 9

Session 5

Identifying Skills for Maintaining Wellness and Building the Wellness Plan

Use This Core Skill for . . .

- All youth to introduce the wellness continuum and the six S's of wellness.
- Please note: When planning for this session, have the youth complete Handout 8.3, Wellness Log, in the preceding week.

Session Objectives

- Identify the wellness continuum.
- Introduce the six S's of wellness.
- Help the youth to develop a Wellness Plan.

Session Checklist

1. Provide the parents with a handout on today's topic while they wait.
2. Set the agenda; elicit the youth's agenda; evidence check (for or against self-belief).
3. Review self-reports (looking for possible residual symptoms).
4. Review the previous session (Did It Stick?, elicit feedback and summary, discuss results of homework/practice, discuss any adherence obstacles).
5. Teach Wellness.

6. How does this skill fit in on the timeline?

7. Perform a homework/adherence check.

8. Elicit feedback and Make It Stick.

INTRODUCTION

After going through items 1–4 of the Session Checklist, begin this part of the session.

> *"Now that your depression is improving, it is a good time to add skills and lifelong strategies to keep you well. What wellness skills do you have now that you want to keep using or use more often?"*

RATIONALE

This is a time in the program when the focus is on maximizing outcomes and maintaining health. To this end, the therapist will identify current skills and strategies that the youth is using to improve and maintain positive mood and identify skills that need to be added.

When people are ill, all focus shifts to the illness and less attention is paid to overall wellness and health. On the illness–wellness continuum, so far this treatment has focused on the illness side and on strategies targeted primarily at reducing depressive symptoms. It is now time to focus on the other side of this continuum—those behaviors and practices that lead to an optimal quality of life.

TEACH/PRACTICE IN SESSION

Wellness Continuum

The final goal of this treatment is to equip the youth with skills for wellness. The youth needs to understand that this treatment does not just strive for the prevention of relapse, but that the end result would be for him or her to "live life to the fullest." Introduce the wellness continuum. Explain the illness–wellness continuum in regard to depression.

> **THERAPIST TIP:** Define continuum as a range where wellness can fluctuate over time. You can be more well or less well; it is not a black and white concept.

"What we have really focused on are skills to reduce depression and depressive symptoms. Now we want to add in skills and tools to increase the amount of time that you are not depressed—these are the positive behaviors and attitudes that keep you healthy and happy! These can be thought of as tools to help extend your periods of wellness.

"Have you ever had an injury, like a sprained ankle? Remember that when you first hurt yourself, you had to stay off of that ankle, and you had to sit out for awhile in sports. Later, when the ankle had healed, you could begin to work on strengthening and conditioning your ankle, making it stronger and more flexible. This should help prevent future injury.

"These wellness skills can be thought of as strengthening your life, helping you to fend off trauma, illness, and stress. When you use these new skills and tools, you will be making yourself more flexible and strong as a person."

The Six S's of Wellness

"Let's look at your 'Wellness Log' together now. What are your thoughts about wellness in your life? What would you like to focus on?"

Review Handout 8.3, Wellness Log, with the youth. Go over each area, identifying and emphasizing areas that the youth already excels in. Validate the youth's strengths and emphasize skills that the youth is already using for wellness. After you've done this, identify any areas of wellness that the youth is willing to work on. In this way, you help the youth to achieve balance in wellness.

This process needs to be collaborative and interactive.

"In this program, there are six general areas of wellness."

The Six S's

1. Self-acceptance (positive self-schema; explanatory style/optimism).
2. Social (social skills, social problem solving).
3. Success (autonomy/mastery).
4. Self-goals (purpose).
5. Spiritual (optimism, gratitude, altruism).
6. Soothing (relaxation) (Ryff & Singer, 1996).

- *Self-acceptance:* Remind the youth of positive/helpful self-statements.

    "Which helpful self-statements are you already using?"

    "Are there some that you would like to increase or practice with more often?"

- *Social:* Social support is particularly important because it is what makes you feel connected in this world, and connections to other people are what make life fun! Consider using Handout 9.2, Who's on Your Team, here.

- *Success:* Having a sense of mastery in some areas of life is important in maintaining wellness. *"Do we notice the good things that happen and our role in them?"* Be aware of attributions for positive events and the importance of building the positive self-schema.

- *Self-Goals:* Having goals gives people hope and a sense of purpose. Discuss with the youth the importance of having short-term goals and long-term goals. Having something to look forward to is an important aspect of keeping up hope and maintaining wellness.

- *Spiritual:* Self-awareness, including recognition of one's values and beliefs and living in conjunction with those values and beliefs, is a key part of wellness. It is also important to respect the views of others (tolerance) and to participate in activities that help others (altruism) in a way that will better connect you to the world around you. Introduce optimism and a hopeful view of the world. Some people get hope from faith: *"Do you have faith (in a higher power? In your values? In yourself?)?"* Revisit the explanatory or attributional style as needed.

- *Soothing:* Stress has detrimental effects on the mind and body. Relaxation is key to maintaining health. It is important to use strategies that are self-soothing. Use the relaxation training and sleep hygiene supplement in the Appendix as needed if this is an area of weakness for the youth. Examples might include taking a bubble bath, listening to relaxing music, and eating a good meal.

SUGGESTED HANDOUTS

✓ The Six S's of Wellness (Handout 9.1)

✓ Who's on Your Team? (Handout 9.2)

✓ Wellness Log (Handout 8.3)

Development of the Wellness Plan

Introduce Handout 9.4, The Plan, collaborating with the youth to complete this plan based on information gathered from Handout 8.3, Wellness Log. The youth may choose to focus on one or two areas of wellness, rather than filling in several categories. Stress that the goal of this activity is to "be the best me."

SUGGESTED HANDOUT

✓ The "Best" Me (Handout 9.3)

✓ The Plan (Handout 9.4)

APPLY TO TIMELINE

"How would these strategies have helped you in the past?"

"How can they help you this week?"

"How can you use them in the future?"

HOMEWORK/PRACTICE

Collaborate with the youth to identify how he or she can use what was learned in this session over the next week. Be specific!
Suggestions include:

1. Have the youth contract to increase one to two wellness strategies during the next week. Brainstorm specific plans to increase the wellness areas (e.g., if a youth wants to increase social wellness, have the youth contract to make plans twice with friends in the upcoming week).

2. Have the youth continue the Wellness Log for the next few weeks to track his or her wellness progress.

3. Come up with some positive self-statements that could be used during the week. Have the youth anticipate situations in the upcoming week where these positive statements could be used. Incorporate positive self statements into self-monitoring and homework assignment.

4. Have the youth pay attention to the good things that happen in the upcoming week. Have the youth practice "taking credit" for these things.

5. Contract with the youth to thank someone who has helped him or her or has done something nice for him or her in the past.

MAKE IT STICK

Have the youth share what he or she learned in the session and list these items on a Make It Stick Post-it note. You can add any additional points to this list. The youth may also give feedback about what was the most helpful from the session. Share what he or she learned about the youth during this session (i.e., reinforce the youth's strengths).

In addition, you can create a postcard to send the youth during the week with the main points from the session. This should help the youth remember to practice what was learned in-session.

Suggested items for the Make It Stick include The Six S's of Wellness (Handout 9.1).

TRANSITIONING TO THE FAMILY SESSION

Discuss the family session with the youth prior to inviting the parents into the session.

First, review what will be discussed in the parent session.

- Work collaboratively with the youth to set a workable agenda for the parent session.

- Determine what issues would be helpful to discuss further.

- Determine any issues that the youth does not want to discuss during the parent session.

IDEAS FOR THE THERAPIST	
Younger youth	**Older youth**
• Use vignettes. • Use drawings or figural representations of wellness strategies. • Use concrete example of behavioral activation. • Teach wellness to parents.	• Use real-life examples.
More behavioral	**More cognitive**
• Assign areas for practice.	• Explanatory style and optimism—help youth identify how these are linked.

- You will want to get the youth's "buy-in" and collaborate with the youth on how this concept may relate to his or her family and be helpful in the youth's treatment.

- Have the youth think about how this new family skill might be applied to the timeline. Consider what the family can do to help support the youth in preventing relapse.

Family Session: Wellness[*]

AGENDA

Collaborate with the family to set an agenda for the family session.

- Check in with the family on any previously assigned homework.

- Elicit feedback on the program and the past week. Continue to gather information on past factors associated with the youth's depression (particularly family factors) and their input on current residual symptoms and anticipated future obstacles (add these to the timeline). Continue to get parent input on treatment goals for the program.

- Elicit any questions parents may have after reviewing the parent handout. An optional agenda item is to have the youth teach the concept of wellness to the parents.

- Discuss the treatment termination plan for the family. Remind the family that three scheduled sessions remain, with optional booster sessions available after that.

- Remember to prioritize the agenda items collaboratively.

TEACH AND PRACTICE

Introduce Wellness

"On the illness–wellness continuum, so far this treatment has focused on the illness side and strategies targeted primarily at reducing depressive symptoms. It is now time to focus on the other side of this continuum—to those behaviors and practices that lead to an optimal quality of life."

---

[*] *Note:* Activities in this family session may be used in the individual session as well.

- Introduce the idea of wellness practices as a protective mechanism to prevent a relapse of depression. Introduce Handout 9.1, the Six S's of Wellness.
- Consider having the youth share his or her wellness plan with the family. What can the family do to support your youth's individual wellness?
- Collaborate with the family to assess the family level of wellness, and possibly develop a family wellness plan, using Handout 9.1. What does the family already do that promotes wellness? What can the family add that will increase wellness? Does the family have enough activities in each of the "S" categories? Do any "S" categories need more? Examples of ways to assess each "S," as well as suggestions for improving an "S" category, are included below.

Self-Acceptance

How does the family contribute to the youth's self-acceptance? How are individual differences valued in the family? What is the view of the family as a whole? What are the family's strengths?

Things to Try

- Reduce negative self-statements and increase positive attributions.
- Develop a family motto or mission statement.
- Have parents serve as coaches to recognize and help correct negative self-statements or negative family attributions.
- Identify and affirm the individual strengths and unique qualities of each family member. Plan ways to acknowledge and celebrate these differences in the home.
- Brainstorm ways that parents can assist the youth in improving the youth's own personal wellness in this area.

Social

How does the family get social support? How can they help their youth have access to more social support?

Things to Try

- Develop a list of family friends and support systems. Complete Handout 9.2, Who's on Your Team?
- Brainstorm ways that parents can assist the youth in improving the youth's own personal wellness in this area.

Success

How does the family succeed? What are you proud of as a family? (Examples include "We keep our home clean," "We take care of our extended family," and "We are good neighbors"). Does the family notice the good things that happen and each member's role in these good things?

Things to Try

- Develop a list of successes that your family has achieved.
- Identify any activities that you would like the family to spend more time on.
- Brainstorm ways that parents can assist the youth in improving the youth's own personal wellness in this area.

Self-Goals

Does the family have any goals? Having goals gives people hope and a sense of purpose.

Things to Try

- Develop a list of goals for the family. What are your goals for this month? For this year? For the next 5 years? Consider tying goals to the family mission statement.
- Discuss the youth's short-term goals and long-term goals with the family. How can the family support these goals?

Spiritual

Self-awareness, including recognition of one's values and beliefs, and living in conjunction with those values and beliefs, is a key part of wellness. It is also important to respect the views of others (tolerance) and to participate in activities that help others (altruism) in a way to better connect to the world around you. Introduce optimism and looking at the world with hope. Some people meet their spiritual needs through faith and/or meditation practices.

Things to Try

- Make a list of altruistic-type activities (e.g., volunteer activities) that the family wishes to try in the next month/year.
- Consider starting a family gratitude journal, where members can add what they are thankful for.

- Consider using a white board or chalkboard, where family members can write statements of gratitude to other family members.
- Have the family practice the "thank a mentor" model, where each member writes an appreciation letter to a personal mentor.
- Brainstorm ways that parents can assist the youth in improving the youth's own personal wellness in this area.

Soothing

How does the family relax together? How do individual members relax?

Things to Try

- Create a list of ways that the family relaxes together. Help the family to expand this list. For example, if a family only relaxes together by watching TV, consider trying other ways to relax, such as taking a walk together, doing a puzzle, or reading together.
- Brainstorm ways that parents can assist the youth in improving the youth's own personal wellness in this area.

SUMMARY AND HOMEWORK/PRACTICE

Summarize the family session.

- Assess the family's understanding of wellness concepts and activities.
- Elicit feedback about the session.
    "How is this relevant to your family's situation?"
    "How can I, as the therapist, be helpful?"
- Have the family summarize the session.

Collaborate to develop a family homework assignment. Homework ideas include:

- Identify the parts of wellness to work on for the week. For example, does the family want to try to work on one "S" per week?
- Contract with the family to do some of the "Things to Try" items discussed previously.

DID IT STICK? (REVIEW QUESTIONS FROM THE SESSION)

1. What is meant by "continuum of wellness"?
2. What are the six S's?
3. How did you improve your overall wellness in the past few weeks?

CASE EXAMPLE: SESSION 5

In Session 5, the therapist and Lily reviewed the FLIP practice activity from the past week. Lily was able to ask a friend to a movie and reported that she had a great time. She had rated her mood before and after the event, and noticed the connection between this social activity and positive mood. Lily reported that her mood rating ranged from 1 to 3 over the past 2 weeks, which was improved from prior weeks. Together, the therapist and Lily examined the thoughts and behaviors that were keeping her mood at this level. She reported being more active and not staying in her room as much, eating dinner with her family at the kitchen table, and accepting her friend's invitation to get frozen yogurt. She also noted that she had been using the thought check skill to develop more helpful thoughts.

The therapist presented the idea and importance of wellness and how being well is connected with our behavior choices, as well as how we view ourselves, our world, and our future. She also explained that wellness skills are helpful in preventing relapse of depression. The six S's of wellness—social activities, soothing activities, self-acceptance, self-goals, success activities, and spiritual activities—were introduced by the therapist. Lily and the therapist reviewed the wellness activity log, noting Lily's wellness strengths and activities she is already doing that might keep her well. In addition, the therapist asked Lily for ideas about what she would like to increase or work on to improve her level of wellness. Lily answered that she would like to focus on increasing social activities, soothing activities, and success activities.

Social activities: Lily's goal is to expand her circle of friends. She was able to identify two additional friends whom she would like to get to know better. Ideas were generated for ways to connect with these friends as well as for ideas of fun things they might do together.

Soothing activities: Lily had very few activities that she found to be relaxing, although she admits that reading is something she finds calming. The therapist asked if she wanted to find out more about soothing activities. The therapist introduced progressive muscle relaxation and deep breathing (see pp. 173–174 in the Appendix for supplemental materials). Together they planned a few practice activities for the upcoming 2 weeks. Lily agreed to practice either deep breathing or progressive muscle relaxation prior to bedtime, as this was a time of worry and stress for her.

Success activities: Lily quickly identified art as something she thinks she is good at; this was highlighted as an area of mastery for Lily. However, she states that she has not been as active in art as she was prior to the onset of her depression. The school has an annual art show each year, and Lily set a goal of entering her work into the show. The immediate plan was to coordinate her participation with the school art teacher and decide on a few projects to work on for submission. In addition, Lily will join her school's art club to increase her opportunities to participate in art projects.

The therapist and Lily planned for the family session. Lily decided to share her planned wellness activities with her parents.

Lily introduced wellness and its relationship to mood and prevention of relapse to her family. The family participated in a family wellness activity. Specifically, they identified areas of the six S's that they would like to improve as a family. They selected spiritual activities and self-goals as areas of wellness to increase.

Spiritual activities: The family identified a desire to do more community service at the local food bank. They decided to schedule to volunteer as a family on Saturday of next week.

Self-goal activities: The family set a family goal of spending more time connecting to one another. They decided to try a family fun night, where each family member would take turns choosing the activity for the week. Lily chose the first activity, which was a Monopoly night. The family agreed to play the game on Thursday night.

THE SIX S's OF WELLNESS

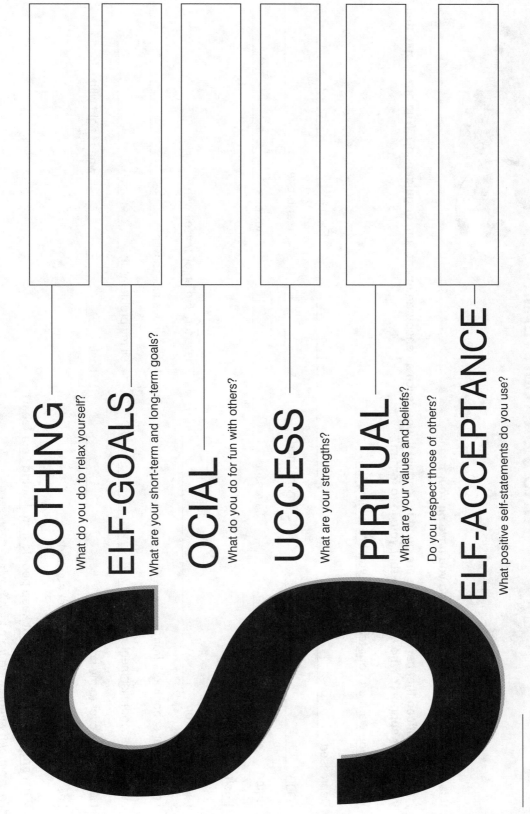

OOTHING

What do you do to relax yourself?

ELF-GOALS

What are your short-term and long-term goals?

OCIAL

What do you do for fun with others?

UCCESS

What are your strengths?

PIRITUAL

What are your values and beliefs?

Do you respect those of others?

ELF-ACCEPTANCE

What positive self-statements do you use?

123

WHO'S ON YOUR TEAM?

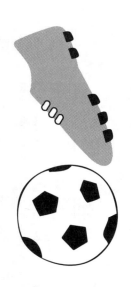

It is important for you to realize who you have on your team.

Have you noticed that certain people are good for certain things (such as encouragement, fun, or guidance)? Who are people that you ask for support? Who are people that you go to for fun?

Who do you want on your team when you are feeling . . .

Depressed _____   Lonely _____   Excited _____

Angry _____   Overwhelmed _____   Heartbroken _____

Bored _____   Distressed _____   Anxious _____

Positions on your team

I seek advice from _____   I have fun and enjoy myself with _____

I get help for schoolwork from _____   I share my success with _____

I share my accomplishments with _____   I tell my problems to _____

I like to invite over to my home _____   I call _____ when I fight with a friend

I go to _____ for support

What are some obstacles that keep people from joining your team?

For example: withdrawing from friends when depressed

_____

THE "BEST" ME

"OLD" ME

Situation	Emotion	Thoughts/Action

"BEST" ME

Emotion	Thoughts/Action

THE PLAN

The goal of this treatment is to keep you from experiencing relapse of depression. A second goal is to improve your life. Below is space for you to fill in your Relapse Prevention Plan and your Wellness Plan.

My Relapse Prevention Plan

My potential triggers (symptoms of lapse)

Helpful skills and techniques that I can use to prevent relapse

_____   _____

_____   _____

_____   _____

_____   _____

My Wellness Plan: The Six S's

Self-Acceptance and Care: I will recognize my strengths and accept them. I will take care of myself by maintaining a healthy diet, exercising, and getting enough sleep.

Soothing: I will regularly take time to relax my mind and body.

Social: I will keep up with the relationships in my life, as I realize that friends and other social support are vital to my well-being.

Success: I understand that it is important for me to keep up with those things that I am good at, as feeling successful improves my mood and self-esteem.

Spiritual: I will behave in ways that are reflective of my values and beliefs, while respecting those of others.

Self-Goals: _____

CHAPTER 10

Sessions 6 and 7

Practice and Application of Core Skills

Use This Core Skill for . . .

- All youth and parents to practice the core skills.
- Use with supplements tailored to help youth apply the core skills to specific common circumstances.

Session Objectives

- Continue to practice using sessions to date.
- Identify strategies for managing identified risk factors for relapse.
- Build on individual and family strengths.
- Identify areas to improve and continue work on Handout 9.4, The Plan (Relapse Prevention Plan and Wellness Plan).

Session Checklist

1. Provide the parents with a handout on today's topic while they wait.
2. Set the agenda; elicit the youth's agenda; evidence check (for or against self-belief).
3. Review self-reports (looking for possible residual symptoms).
4. Review the previous session (Did It Stick?, elicit feedback and summary, discuss results of homework/practice, discuss any adherence obstacles).

Note. Sessions 6 and 7 can be individual or conjoint sessions.

5. Teach new skills.

6. How does this skill fit in on the timeline?

7. Perform homework/adherence check.

8. Elicit feedback and Make It Stick.

INTRODUCTION

After going through items 1–4 of the Session Checklist, begin this part of the session.

> *"In this part of the treatment, we will continue to practice and apply the core skills of behavioral coping, cognitive restructuring, problem solving, and wellness to different situations and examples from your life."*

RATIONALE

Learning a new skill and making it part of everyday life take practice. As such, we want to continue to highlight skills added to the timeline. Similarly, we want to build on the skills the youth already has—perhaps increasing those times and experiences of positive mood or wellness.

> *"How have you used skills this week to manage your mood?"*
>
> *"Are you noticing when good things happen?"*

THERAPIST TIP: Continue to look for attributions related to both positive and negative events.

TEACH

Review the core skill (selected for review) and apply to the issue.

PRACTICE IN SESSION

Use the new skill with a past or an anticipated problem to help the youth practice skills application. It is important to use items on the agenda when possible. Remember, using "real life" to practice makes the skills more useful and easy to remember and use again!

Role-play with the youth using the new skill as needed.

OPTIONAL ACTIVITY: **Looking Forward**

For example, if the youth's negative self-belief is "I am unlovable," think of times that this belief could be activated in the future.

> *"We've been working so hard on making this negative self-belief not a problem anymore. What are some situations ahead where you are at risk or vulnerable?"*

> What if the youth is not asked to the prom? What would your thoughts "look like" in this scenario? What could you do to change these thoughts? How would this affect your mood and behavior?

APPLY TO TIMELINE

In this phase of treatment, focus on the timeline. The main goal is to consolidate use of the core skills, so work with any examples or issues from the timeline, as well as those brought in by the youth.

> *"How would these strategies have helped you in the past?"*

> *"How can they help you this week?"*

> *"How can you use them in the future?"*

HOMEWORK/PRACTICE

Collaborate with the youth to identify how he or she can use what was learned in this session over the next week. Be specific!

Collaborate on a way to practice the skill: Anticipate obstacles and find solutions. How might the youth let you know how it worked before the next meeting?

MAKE IT STICK

Have the youth share what he or she learned in the session and list these items on a Make It Stick Post-it note. You can add any additional points to this list. The youth may also give feedback about what was the most helpful from the session. Share what you learned about the youth during this session (i.e., reinforce the youth's strengths).

In addition, you can create a postcard to send the youth during the week with the main points from the session. This should help the youth remember to practice what was learned in-session.

IDEAS FOR THE THERAPIST	
Younger youth	**Older youth**
• Use vignettes. • Have youth teach parent the skill at end of session/ parent check-in.	• Use real-life examples. • Be very specific in how the skill could be applied in the youth's life.
More behavioral	**More cognitive**
• Use role play and behavioral rehearsal.	• Anticipate obstacles ahead by planning out the practice of the skill.

Suggested items for the Make It Stick include:

• Strategies or acronyms from the supplement.

• Application of skill to a specific, personal example.

Family Check-In

Check in with the family to see how the youth was able to participate in wellness activities since the previous session.

DID IT STICK?

Review the previous session. Use the questions to assess this, depending on the skill supplement used.

CASE EXAMPLE: SESSIONS 6 AND 7

At the beginning of Session 6, the therapist and Lily reviewed wellness skills. Lily reported that she enjoyed the game night and that she had tried the breathing strategies during the past week.

When setting the agenda, Lily reported that her mood was a little worse over the past 2 weeks. She attributed this drop in mood to her sister getting invited to a party. Lily's not being included brought up some old, unhelpful thinking patterns of not being good enough and not fitting in. Together, the therapist and Lily were able to tie her decreased mood to her comparisons to her sister and her tendency to judge herself as being a "loser." Using the thought check skill, the therapist and Lily examined these thoughts and generated more helpful thoughts. Lily wrote these helpful thoughts on a notecard to keep in her room.

In addition, the FLIP skill was reviewed to take another look at what Lily could do to widen her circle of friends. Since one of Lily's goals was to join the art club, the therapist asked if there were any people in art that Lily might want to get to know better. She stated that her school had an after-school art program where students are able to work on projects collectively. The therapist used the social support supplement to help Lily plan how she might increase her social network through the art program. Lily created a plan to consult with her art teacher to see if she might participate. The therapist asked Lily to re-rate her mood after the session. She rated a significant improvement in mood, noting that these plans made her feel more hopeful. The plans and goals discussed in these sessions were added to Handout 9.4, The Plan, which includes the wellness activities and relapse prevention skills.

Session 7 followed a structure similar to Session 6, with Lily and the therapist collaborating to review and practice skills as needed. Lily reported on her mood, which was much improved from the last session. She attributed this improvement to her ability to join in on the collective art project through art club and to feeling overall more positive about her social life. She reported using more helpful thoughts and self-talk strategies when she finds herself comparing herself to her sister ("We both have different strengths; comparisons are not helpful.").

CHAPTER 11

Session 8

Relapse Prevention Plan and Wellness Plan

Use This Core Skill for . . .

- All youth and parents after primary skills have been identified in the RP-CBT program—prior to booster sessions.

Session Objectives

- Assist the youth in developing a Relapse Prevention Plan.
- Identify lapse and relapse and collaborate on when to seek help (signs and symptoms of relapse).
- Anticipate upcoming stressors and apply skills from the Relapse Prevention Plan.
- Confirm/modify the Relapse Prevention Plan, including the parents' role in the plan.
- Help the youth to identify the Wellness Plan (the six S's).

Session Checklist

1. Provide the parents with a handout on today's topic while they wait.
2. Set the agenda; elicit the youth's agenda; evidence check (for or against self-belief).

3. Review self-reports (looking for possible residual symptoms).

4. Review the previous session (Did It Stick?, elicit feedback and summary, discuss results of homework/practice, discuss any adherence obstacles).

5. Develop the Relapse Prevention Plan and Wellness Plan.

6. How does this skill fit in on the timeline?

7. Perform homework/adherence check.

8. Elicit feedback and Make It Stick.

9. Invite parents into the session to participate in development of The Plan (Handout 11.2).

INTRODUCTION

After going through items 1–4 of the Session Checklist, begin this part of the session.

> *"Well, we have finally reached the end of the road for this treatment! However, the road does not stop here; it continues with you being the one in the driver's seat. It is my hope that you feel proud of all that you have accomplished in this treatment."*

For older youth, use the metaphor of being your own therapist.

Refer to the youth's timeline, pointing out the bank of skills that has been added throughout the course of treatment.

> *"Today's focus will be on the last part of this timeline: the future. I would like for us to talk about your personal Relapse Prevention Plan. I also want to discuss your Wellness Plan because I want you to not only keep from having a relapse, but to also live life to the fullest!"*

RATIONALE

This session is the culmination of the continuation phase of the treatment. At this point, the timeline will be complete, and this timeline will include several skills that the youth has learned to use. The major goal of this final session is to consolidate the Relapse Prevention Plan that has been developed throughout the therapy and to introduce the idea of the Wellness Plan, which aims toward continued optimal quality of life. It is important to remind the youth (and his or her family) that additional sessions are available as needed. Collaborating on the signs and symptoms of relapse for this youth is essential, and knowing how to get support and seek appropriate help is an important goal of this session.

TEACH/PRACTICE IN SESSION

Identify Lapse, Relapse, and When to Seek Treatment

Introduce the term *lapse* to the youth. A lapse is a temporary return of a symptom or cluster of symptoms. Lapses are common and are not necessarily a cause for alarm.

LAPSE DOES NOT EQUAL RELAPSE! The challenge with a lapse is to keep it from becoming a relapse. The youth has been equipped with skills he or she can use to do just this.

"One way to prevent relapse is to monitor yourself in the present—your mood, your thoughts, your behaviors, and your feelings. You will have lapses of some of your symptoms. A lapse could be a sad afternoon, a couple of days where you feel irritable and stressed, or even a week where you feel anxious. None of these are necessarily reasons to be nervous about a relapse. It is important to monitor these feelings and use the skills that you have learned in this program to help you maintain your overall mood and stay well."

SUGGESTED HANDOUTS

✓ Lapse versus Relapse (Handout 11.1)

✓ The Plan (Handout 11.2)

✓ The "Best" Me (Handout 11.3)

Anticipate Upcoming Stressors

Another way to prevent relapse is to anticipate any upcoming stressors and to be proactive in maintaining your mood during this time. Remind the youth of the times during the treatment that you have applied the skill to the past, present, and future. This is comparable to application of skills to the future.

"Remember each week how we applied the new skill to your past, present, and future? Well, thinking about the future is an important way to prevent relapse as well. The more you can anticipate the 'bumps in the road,' the easier it will be for you to slow down, adjust your thinking, and figure out which skills to use prior to those stressors."

Relapse Prevention Plan

This plan has been the focus throughout this treatment. At this point, the youth should have a completed timeline, with several skills (i.e., "tools in the backpack") available for use. Consider reviewing each skill using the handout given to parents for today's session. Using the timeline, have the youth complete the Relapse Prevention Plan part of Handout 11.2, The Plan.

Does the plan need to be modified in any way? Anticipate the obstacles ahead using the skills on the plan. Are there additional skills to add or change in any way?

Wellness Plan

The final goal of this treatment is to equip the youth with skills for wellness. The youth needs to understand that we don't just strive for the prevention of relapse, but that we would like for him or her to "live life to the fullest."

Complete the final wellness plan that was started in Session 7.

APPLY TO TIMELINE

"How would these strategies have helped you in the past?"

"How can they help you this week?"

"How can you use them in the future?"

Connect Handout 11.2 to the timeline, using the skills and strengths from the timeline in the plans.

HOMEWORK/PRACTICE

Work out a method for self-monitoring with the youth. Consider using the metaphor of "being one's own therapist."

Suggestions include:

1. Contract with the youth to follow the Relapse Prevention and Wellness Plan until you see him or her again.

2. Develop positive/helpful self-statements that could be used during the week. Have the youth anticipate situations in the upcoming week when these positive statements could be used. Incorporate positive self-statements into self-monitoring and homework assignments.

3. Have the youth pay attention to the good things that happen in the upcoming week. Have the youth practice "taking credit" for these things.

MAKE IT STICK

Have the youth share what he or she learned in the session and list these items on a Make It Stick Post-it note. You can add any additional points to this list. The youth may also give feedback about what was the most helpful from the session. Share what you learned about the youth during this session (i.e., reinforce the youth's strengths).

In addition, you can create a postcard to send the youth during the week with the main points from the session. This should help the youth remember to practice what was learned in-session.

Suggested items for the Make It Stick include:

- Favorite skills learned in this treatment
- The Plan (Handout 11.2), as a large Post-it note

TRANSITIONING TO THE FAMILY SESSION

Discuss the family session with the youth prior to inviting parents into the session.
First, review what will be discussed in the parent session.

- Work collaboratively with the youth to set a workable agenda for the parent session.
- Have the youth identify the role he or she wants the parents to play in the Relapse Prevention Plan and Wellness Plan.

IDEAS FOR THE THERAPIST	
Younger youth	**Older youth**
• Role-play specific events or situations that include anticipated obstacles ahead. Have the youth demonstrate how he or she will manage the obstacle.	• Use real-life examples. • Have the youth go back to the timeline and imagine him- or herself in old/past upsetting situations; now using new skills, how would he or she handle the situation?
More behavioral	**More cognitive**
• What are the skills that will keep me well? • What should I do when I feel sad? Where do I get support? Who do I have on my team—do different people play different positions? • If I do a think check, what will I be looking for? • Will my Relapse Prevention Plan help me if I look at it? Where should I keep it?	• What are the unhelpful thoughts to look out for? What are the red flag words? What are the red flag emotions? What helpful thoughts or self statements are key in my Relapse Prevention Plan?

- Determine what issues would be helpful to discuss further.
- Determine any issues that the youth does not want to discuss during the parent session.

Family Session: Relapse Prevention and Wellness Plan

AGENDA

Collaborate with the family to set an agenda for the family session.

- Check in with the family on any previously assigned homework.
- Elicit feedback on the program and the past week.
- Elicit any questions parents may have after reviewing the parent handout.
- With the youth's permission and when appropriate, get the family's input on the youth's relapse prevention and wellness plan.
- Remember to prioritize the agenda items collaboratively.

TEACH AND PRACTICE

Explain the rationale for bringing together the two major pieces of this treatment: Relapse Prevention and Wellness.

- The youth should be able to present his or her ideas about how parents can support his or her Relapse Prevention Plan and Wellness Plan.
- Be sure to check in with the family on the Family Wellness Plan. Review with the family the use of optional booster sessions and how this will be negotiated (e.g., will you schedule these sessions, or will the family call if needed?).

SUMMARY AND HOMEWORK/PRACTICE

Summarize the family session.

- Assess the family's understanding of the overall treatment and the future use of booster sessions.
- Elicit feedback about the session.

    "How is this relevant to your family's situation?"

    "How can I, as the therapist, be helpful?"

- Have the family summarize the session.

CASE EXAMPLE: SESSION 8

After setting the agenda and checking in on past practice assignments and mood, the therapist and Lily worked on Handout 11.2, The Plan, to summarize Lily's progress to date. Lily was able to identify several symptoms of lapse that would alert her to use the skills she has learned in the session. For example, when she notices that she has low energy or motivation, she could use one of her behavioral coping skills (Expend energy: riding her bike). When she notices feeling sad, she could use a distraction skill or do a thought check. "Stress" was added to her list of symptoms to watch for. Lily described how she could use the FLIP skill to make a list of things to try to reduce stress. She also noted that deep breathing and reading help her relax. Additionally, Lily said that she plans to continue monitoring for unhelpful thoughts, as doing this would be important in staying well. The therapist and Lily reviewed her coping card of helpful thoughts. They added additional thoughts to this list and referenced it on the timeline and The Plan.

The Wellness Plan component of The Plan built upon what was developed in Session 5. In addition to the social, soothing, and success goals from Session 5, Lily added self-acceptance and self-care activities. She created a weekly exercise schedule, a routine sleep schedule (see sleep supplement), and planned to improve her eating habits by increasing protein and decreasing sugar and soda. She also added that she and her family began volunteering in church outreach activities, which she found to be enjoyable. She added this activity to her own list of spiritual wellness goals.

Once Lily and the therapist completed The Plan, Lily's parents joined the session to review The Plan and their role in supporting Lily's continued wellness.

LAPSE VERSUS RELAPSE

Lapses are normal:

For me, a lapse might look like . . .

_____

_____

_____

_____

_____

A relapse might look like . . .

_____

_____

_____

_____

_____

Lapse does not = Relapse!!!

Things I can do when I have a lapse are . . .

_____

_____

_____

_____

_____

_____

_____

THE PLAN

The goal of this treatment is to keep you from experiencing relapse of depression. A second goal is to improve your life. Below is space for you to fill in your Relapse Prevention Plan and your Wellness Plan.

My Relapse Prevention Plan

My potential triggers (symptoms of lapse)   Helpful skills and techniques that I can use to prevent relapse

_____   _____

_____   _____

_____   _____

_____   _____

_____   _____

My Wellness Plan: The Six S's

Self-Acceptance and Care: I will recognize my strengths and accept them. I will take care of myself by maintaining a healthy diet, exercising, and getting enough sleep.

Soothing: I will regularly take time to relax my mind and body.

Social: I will keep up with the relationships in my life, as I realize that friends and other social support are vital to my well-being.

Success: I understand that it is important for me to keep up with those things that I am good at, as feeling successful improves my mood and self-esteem.

Spiritual: I will behave in ways that are reflective of my values and beliefs, while respecting those of others.

Self-Goals: _____

THE "BEST" ME

"OLD" ME

"BEST" ME

Situation	Emotion	Thoughts/Action	Emotion	Thoughts/Action

CHAPTER 12

Graduation Session and Booster Sessions

GRADUATION SESSION (MAY OCCUR IN SESSION 9, 10, OR 11)

The youth should be made aware of the end of the treatment ahead of the last session (recommended to be discussed and scheduled two to three sessions before the final session). This is an important session to review what the youth has learned in the treatment and to identify what has been most helpful to him or her.

Depending on the developmental level of the child, you can prepare a certificate of completion, a graduation document, or some sort of badge/ribbon representing the completion of the program. For all children, a notebook or binder of the handouts should be prepared ahead that contains the work that they did during the treatment. This binder can serve both as a resource and as a symbolic marker of the end of treatment. The binder should include copies of postcards and Make It Stick notes. The timeline should be included in the binder and will be an important tool for identifying signs and symptoms to monitor for signs of relapse. A certificate can be used for the cover, if appropriate. Collaborate with the youth to summarize the most important points and/or helpful skills while he or she reviews the contents of the binder.

Some children might benefit from metaphors such as becoming your own "coach" or "therapist." They can be encouraged to anticipate problems and/or symptoms and to verbalize their strategy for managing them. The workbook might serve as a "playbook" for reference in determining strategies for preventing relapse.

In this session, it will be important to also review the Relapse Prevention Plan and Wellness Plan with the youth. The mood and tone of the session should be celebratory, and the family should be included in the final part of the session to review these plans and to finalize their role in supporting the child's maintenance of gains.

BOOSTER SESSIONS: SESSIONS 9–11 (MONTHLY FOR 3 MONTHS; INDIVIDUAL OR CONJOINT AS NEEDED)

Use these booster sessions to . . .

- Conduct a graduation session with the youth (see page 144).
- Consolidate skills learned.
- Review skills already taught.
- Add additional skills as needed.

Session Objectives

- Review skills previously learned and evaluate their importance in the Relapse Prevention Plan.
- Identify new skills that may be helpful to the youth.
- Teach the skill.
- Identify lapse, relapse, and when to call.
- Anticipate upcoming stressors and apply new skill and skills already learned (in tool box) from the Relapse Prevention Plan.
- Tie new skills to the timeline.
- Add new skills to the Relapse Prevention and Wellness plans.
- Anticipate obstacles ahead, develop strategies for reducing risk for relapse, and identify additional wellness strategies.
- Look for attributions of positive events and ways to build a positive self-schema.
- Plan practice of skill.

Session Checklist

1. Provide the parents with a handout on today's topic while they wait.
2. Set the agenda; elicit the youth's "stuff"; evidence check (for or against self-belief).
3. Review self-reports (looking for possible residual symptoms).
4. Review the previous session (Did It Stick?, elicit feedback and summary, discuss results of homework/practice, discuss any adherence obstacles).

5. Review or teach skills.

6. How does this skill fit in on the timeline?

7. Perform homework/adherence check.

8. Elicit feedback and Make It Stick.

CASE EXAMPLE: GRADUATION SESSION

In preparation for this session, the therapist compiled the copies of worksheets, Post-it notes, and postcards that had been generated during the RP-CBT treatment. These copies were placed in a binder for easy review in the graduation session.

The session started with a mood check and agenda setting. Lily's mood had remained stable, and she had few items for the agenda. She has been active socially and has maintained an average mood rating of 2. She reported on the changes that she has made that have been positive, including participating in the art show, hanging with some new friends from the art program, and getting along better with her sister. The therapist decided to use Handout 11.3, The "Best" Me, to visually demonstrate the significant changes that Lily has made over the course of treatment.

The therapist and Lily reviewed the skills she learned in each session, looking at the binder and reflecting on their work together. They discussed anticipated obstacles ahead and how Lily might use her skills to address these challenges. Lily discussed feeling nervous about eighth grade, as some of her current friends were going to a different school. Lily and the therapist discussed how Lily could use the thought check skill and the FLIP problem-solving skill to plan ahead for keeping in touch with those friends and making some new friends. They also reviewed how she could use behavioral coping skills to help her mood on days when she especially missed her old friends.

Lily and the therapist collaborated to develop a plan for how Lily might ask for support if she notices a change in her mood. The therapist used Handout 11.1, Lapse versus Relapse, to help Lily identify areas to watch for (e.g., isolating herself in her room, being more irritable at home, and wanting to take more naps), as well as plans for managing these symptoms when they arise. They also reviewed the completed timeline together, noting all of Lily's hard work. The concept of being your own therapist was discussed, as well as how this might work for Lily.

The therapist praised Lily's efforts in therapy and reviewed her progress throughout treatment. During the family session, the parents provided input on Lily's progress. Lily shared The Plan with her parents. The family again reviewed important symptoms to monitor for relapse, such as sleep and irritability. Lily and her family identified specific ways that the family could support Lily, including encouraging her participation in art and social activities, as well as continuing to engage in family activities such as game night and volunteering.

CHAPTER 13

Future Directions

RP-CBT has now been tested through two randomized controlled trials (Kennard et al., 2006, 2014). This book has described both the treatment itself and its use as part of a sequential treatment strategy approach to preventing relapse in youth with major depressive disorder. Sequencing treatments, adding CBT after response to antidepressant medication as opposed to continuation treatment with pharmacotherapy alone, can significantly reduce the risk of relapse and lengthen the time to relapse in youth being treated for depression (Kennard et al., 2014).

The optimal timing of adding CBT is still not well understood. The National Institute for Health and Care Excellence (NICE) guidelines indicate that youth with depression should be treated with CBT as a first-line treatment; however, acute-phase CBT, at least in more severely depressed populations, does not compare as favorably to antidepressant medication or combination treatments (TADS, 2004). In the Treatment for Adolescents with Depression Study (TADS), remission rates to CBT were not comparable to medication until 18 to 24 weeks into treatment (TADS, 2004). RP-CBT has been used as an effective continuation-phase treatment strategy. It will be important in the future to determine the optimal timing of the onset of adding CBT in continuation treatment. Furthermore, whether a different treatment modality could be used for the acute phase is worthy of future examination.

Sequencing effective monotherapies improves outcomes in youth with depression and may be a way to optimize both medication and CBT treatment effects. The RP-CBT strategy is efficient in that it reduces the number of CBT sessions required for positive outcomes (from 12–16 sessions to 8–11) (Kennard et al., 2008a) and thus reduces the burden of time and cost. In addition, RP-CBT emphasizes reducing

145

residual symptoms, preventing relapse, and promoting wellness. Similar to adult studies (Fava et al., 2004), continuation strategies focused on well-being may protect against relapse in depression.

What is unknown is which components of RP-CBT were most helpful in reducing symptoms and promoting wellness. Furthermore, matching the treatment components to specific patient characteristics might increase the efficiency of treatment and result in improved outcomes. Future studies of RP-CBT could help us better understand which components are most essential.

Continuation-phase strategies designed to reduce the high rates of relapse in depressed youth have an important public health impact. RP-CBT offers one approach to protecting depressed youth from relapse and recurrence of symptoms. It is important that we move beyond the short-term goal of just getting children well to the longer-term goal of promoting and maintaining wellness in youth.

Supplemental Materials

Evidenced-based treatments typically are guided by the treatment manuals developed from the clinical trials establishing their efficacy. Although these manuals yield important procedures and guidelines for treating illness, inevitably there are unexpected obstacles or specific situations that are not addressed in the manual. In this appendix, we describe the frequent challenges that we experienced in providing RP-CBT to teens recovering from depression.

Although treating depression is the primary target for RP-CBT, teens and families can present with a variety of issues that may not be easily addressed with the core skills presented in this treatment approach. It is important for the therapist to recognize these issues and to use a flexible approach to managing them as they arise. In the designing of the original manual, the therapy development team identified several potential obstacles that can be presented in treatment. Supplemental materials were created to serve as useful tools for the therapist in addressing these issues. In this chapter, we provide those materials that were used most frequently in the clinical trial. The supplemental materials are presented in an easy-to-use, brief format that provides the therapist with suggested language and skills to utilize in the treatment sessions. Although the core of this treatment is presented in the previous session chapters, these supplements are designed to be used in conjunction with the core skills of RP-CBT.

Adherence Supplement

Use This Supplement for . . .

- A youth who has difficulty completing collaborative homework or practice assignments outside of the therapy session.
- A youth who has limited motivation to participate in therapy.
- A youth who has unrealistic or perfectionistic goals regarding his or her treatment progress.

SKILLS TO CONSIDER

- Cognitive restructuring and automatic thoughts
- Problem solving

STRATEGIES TO TRY FOR INCOMPLETE HOMEWORK

1. LISTEN! Validate the youth's feelings about the importance/relevance of homework.
2. Cognitive restructuring: Explore the youth's thoughts about homework.
   - Identify unhelpful thoughts.
   - Assess for hopelessness.
   - Demonstrate how thoughts influence actions (e.g., think it won't work → don't do it → impact on future → they do not meet their goals/limited change).
   - Collaborate to develop alternative thoughts or more "helpful" thoughts.
3. Maintain a nonjudgmental approach when addressing noncompliance in therapy.
4. Nonadherence with homework is not uncommon in teens; assess if the youth understands the rationale for practice and/or needs more structure to complete homework.
5. Get the teen's input. The youth may understand the homework but not understand how it is relevant to his or her stated treatment goals. Brainstorm with the youth on how practicing outside of the session could be more helpful or relevant.
6. Problem solving: Investigate what barriers prevented doing the homework.
   - Explore barriers to homework.
   - Problem-solving approach.

> *"Do you remember what 'experiment activity' (homework) we talked about your doing this week?"*
>
> *"What is your understanding of why we decided to do this 'experiment' (homework)?"*
>
> *"Did/do you have time to complete the activity?"*
>
> *"Let's try to pick a specific time to do the activity."*
>
> *"What do you think prevented you from completing the homework?"*
>
> *"Can you think of any solutions to those obstacles?"*

- Assess with the youth the likelihood of completing the assignment. Ask the youth what is the percentage from 1 to 100 that he or she will be likely to complete the homework. Then ask the youth how you could help increase the likelihood that he or she would be able to complete the assignment. For example, you could ask, "How could we increase the likelihood by 10%, and what if we wanted to increase it by 20%?"

7. Examine other areas of functioning.

- Explore if the youth has trouble with adherence in daily functioning such as school work, chores, or taking medication.

- Try to assess if the trouble involves just therapy homework or if the youth has difficulty completing school homework as well. If the nonadherence is limited to therapy work, then motivation to attend therapy, obstacles to complete homework, and expectations of therapy should be addressed. However, if the youth has trouble with other tasks as well (school homework, chores, money management, etc.), then it may be important to teach the youth skills to aid in organizing and planning ahead.

THERAPIST TIP: Important Factors for Collaborative Decisions on Homework

1. Review the rationale/goals.

   a. Tie homework to the timeline and the Relapse Prevention Plan.

   b. Help the teen identify the relevance of the practice to his or her goals.

2. Collaborate with the youth to create homework assignments.

3. Confirm that the youth understands the instructions and homework assignment.

4. Investigate possible barriers to completing homework.

   a. Rate the likelihood that the homework will be done as assigned.

5. Practice homework in-session.

STRATEGIES TO TRY TO ADDRESS PERFECTIONISM

1. Warn against perfectionism and introduce a *continuum of progress*. Some progress is better than no progress. For example, the youth will not go from making C's to making A's overnight.

2. Examine the beliefs of perfectionism regarding treatment.

   - *"Where are you on the continuum of wellness?"*

   - *"How will you know when you are moving forward on this continuum?"*

   - *"What specific things will improve when you move forward [e.g., A's on report card, lots of friends]?"*

SUGGESTED HANDOUT

✓ FLIP the Problem (Handout 8.1)

Anxiety Supplement

Use This Supplement for . . .

- A youth who reports residual symptoms of anxiety in social situations, in the school environment, or in other situations.

SKILLS TO CONSIDER

- Cognitive restructuring and automatic thoughts
- Relaxation training and sleep hygiene supplement

STRATEGIES TO TRY

1. Elicit situations where the youth has felt anxious. The therapist will likely have examples from previous sessions to help the youth with this task. Consider introducing the idea of anxiety on a continuum.

   - Help the youth to identify an anxiety-provoking situation that occurs most frequently or that is the most intense/maladaptive. Past Mood Logs may help with this.

2. Recognize the emotional, physiological, and cognitive indicators of anxiety.

   > *"Now I want you to think back to a time when you were in that situation and feeling very nervous. Put yourself back in that situation. I want you to try to remember everything: where you were, who was there, what time it was, what was happening around you, as much as you can remember.*
   >
   > *"Now describe how you are feeling (nervous, anxious, stressed out—use the youth's language). What are you doing? What is happening in your body? Does your stomach hurt, is your heart racing, are your palms sweaty, are you feeling light-headed?*
   >
   > *"What thoughts are going through your head?"*

   - Link the thoughts to the emotion of fear or anxiety. If the thought is altered, how does that impact the intensity of the emotion? Help the youth generate more helpful thoughts for situations when he or she experiences anxiety.

OPTIONAL ACTIVITY

If the youth is having trouble identifying thoughts, behaviors, and feelings from his or her own situations, it may be helpful to use an example. "You are walking down an unfamiliar street in a neighborhood. You begin to hear footsteps behind you."
    Identify the emotion, thought, and behavior.

      Feeling: Nervous, scared.

      Thought: "Someone is following me; someone may hurt me."

      Behavior: Run away or walk faster.

"Now, imagine the same situation (same sounds, same street, etc.) and the footsteps belong to a person who has picked up an important notebook that you had unknowingly dropped on the street.
    "What has changed? Your interpretation of the situation has changed."

This is an example of "change the thought, change the mood."
    Explore this further by changing the thought again. For example, a person has a surprise package for you. The thought would change again, with the resulting emotion being joy.

---

5. Problem solving: Discuss the pros and cons of avoidance. Make decisions about which situations should be avoided and which ones could be addressed using new skills.

   • Talk about any situations that the youth may have avoided to alleviate anxiety.

      "When we avoid the situations that make us nervous, it may help in the short term, but in the long run, it makes us forget the skills that we have to help us cope. You have learned (will learn) several skills that can help you cope with anxiety feelings and false alarms."

   THERAPIST TIP: Consider exposure techniques for those situations that cannot be avoided. For example, if a youth has anxiety about speaking in class, then use graded exposure techniques for practice assignments. Explore the thoughts surrounding this anxiety.

6. Discuss skills that the youth has mastered that have increased his or her competency in social situations (interpersonal skills, assertiveness training, relaxation training).

7. Behavioral coping, positive self-talk, and problem solving: Introduce the youth to the BREAK strategy.

   • **B:** Believe in the ability to cope.

   • **R:** Relaxation techniques.

   • **E:** Evaluate the situation.

- **A:** Alarm—false or real?
- **K:** Keep your cool.
  - Believe in your ability to cope. Encourage the youth to use positive self-talk to create a sense of hopefulness around the concept of coping with anxiety.
  - Relaxation techniques. See the supplement below on relaxation strategies. Techniques that have been effective thus far for the youth, such as deep breathing or progressive muscle relaxation, should be applied here.
  - Evaluate the situation. Work with the youth to identify the source of his or her anxiety and the automatic negative thoughts that contribute to the feeling of anxiety.
  - Alarm—false or real? *"One great way to put those false alarms in their place is to practice all of the skills that you have learned. False alarms make it very easy for us to forget that we have these skills."*
  - Keep your cool. Emphasize the importance of practice.

    "Practicing the skills now will enable you to tolerate stressful situations in the future. In other words, practicing the skills now will help you to 'keep your cool' and have more confidence to manage your anxiety during an actual anxiety-provoking situation."

Create a homework assignment for the week ahead, giving the youth the opportunity to use the BREAK strategy. Stress to the youth that some discomfort is normal when facing anxiety and that it will likely be uncomfortable to complete the assignment. Work with the youth to find a task that will be comfortable enough to tolerate. In addition, work with the youth to find a reward or self-soothing activity to do after completing the task. Elicit expected outcomes of the task and work through them together. Consider using Coping Cards with helpful counterthoughts.

> **THERAPIST TIP:** It is very important to evaluate the likelihood that the youth will do the assignment. It is most important that he or she does not avoid practice. Work with the youth to determine a homework assignment that is feasible. Completion is the most important thing. Refer to the adherence supplement for more tips on homework.

> **SUGGESTED HANDOUT**
> ✓ Take a BREAK (Handout A.1)

Assertiveness Supplement

Use This Supplement for . . .

- A youth who has difficulty with negotiation, feeling that he or she never gets what he or she wants.

- A youth who has difficulty compromising in family, social, and academic settings.

- A family that has difficulty with problem solving and communication.

- A youth who has trouble expressing thoughts, feelings, and/or beliefs in a direct, honest, and appropriate way in certain situations, such as saying "no" to a friend, asking for an unreasonable favor, having trouble giving or receiving a compliment, being afraid to ask for help, or feeling that his or her life is controlled by others.

SKILLS TO CONSIDER

- Cognitive restructuring and automatic thoughts

STRATEGIES TO TRY

1. Cognitive restructuring.
    - Elicit situations in which the youth has had difficulty being assertive and work with the youth to identify the automatic negative thought(s) that contributes to this lack of assertiveness. It is very important to determine exactly what the youth is afraid of in situations that he or she is less assertive. Once the automatic negative thought is identified, work with the youth to do a "thought check" to evaluate the thought and restructure it to make it more helpful.

    - Explore recent situations involving interpersonal conflict; identify the youth's role in the conflict and look for skills that may be helpful that have already been reviewed, such as unhelpful thoughts or problem solving.

    - Identify the automatic negative thoughts and cognitive distortions that contribute to the conflict. Difficulties in compromising can be related to automatic thoughts or cognitive distortions.

    - Using examples from the role plays or examples the youth has brought up earlier in treatment, you may identify automatic thoughts or distortions that may get in the way of listening or of compromising.

2. Teach the youth to communicate his or her needs in a clear manner while still respecting his or her rights and feelings, as well as the rights and feelings of others. Introduce the WIN strategy for being assertive:

- **W:** Wait and listen to what the other person is saying.
  - It is important to acknowledge the other person's perspective, even though the youth may not agree with the stance of the other person. One way that the youth can show that he or she is listening would be to reflect back on what the youth heard the other person say.
- **I:** Use "I" statements.
  - *"An 'I' message is a good way to let people know what you are thinking. It is made up of three parts."*

    Behavior—What is it, exactly, that the other person has done or is doing?

    Feelings—What *effect* does the other person's *behavior* have on your *feelings*?

    Effect—What is happening because of the other person's behavior?

    By using this kind of message, you are giving another person complete information, leaving no room for second-guessing or doubt—for example: "When you come late to the meeting [behavior], I feel angry [feelings] because we have to repeat information that the rest of us have already discussed [effect]."
  - Use "I," not "You."

    Example:

    "You always interrupt my stories!" (aggressive response)

    "I would like to tell my story without being interrupted." (assertive)
  - Express thoughts, feelings, and opinions reflecting ownership.

    Example:

    "He makes me angry." (denying ownership of feelings)

    "I get angry when he breaks his promises." (assertive and taking ownership of own feelings)
- **N:** Negotiate a compromise to get what you want. Use the FLIP skill and emphasize the importance of waiting and listening to help move to compromise.

3. Help the youth distinguish between passive, aggressive, and assertive responses.
- *Passive responses* fail to express honest feelings, thoughts, and beliefs. If feelings are expressed, they are expressed in an apologetic way that others can easily disregard. This style allows a person to avoid conflict or confrontation or give into the pressure of the situation. It often leaves the person feeling weak and powerless. Sometimes a passive response is actually not responding at all.

  Example: Saying it is okay, even though you feel your viewpoint was not respected.
- *Aggressive responses* are responses in which the person stands up for his or

her rights in a way that is inappropriate and may be perceived as hostile or sarcastic. Aggression offends the rights or feelings of other people and often does not resolve the issues.

> *Example:* Blaming a friend for asking out the person you like by saying, "You don't care about me, you are trying to hurt me on purpose!"

- *Assertive responses* acknowledge personal rights but also acknowledge the rights of other people. Assertive people are able to state their request in a way that does not invalidate the rights of others. These people are able to recognize the other person's perspective, in addition to stating their own viewpoint.

> *Example:* "I understand that you like this boy/girl, but it hurts my feelings that you are asking him/her out."

SUGGESTED HANDOUTS

✓ Thought Check (Handout 7.3)

✓ WIN (Handout A.2)

Anhedonia Supplement

Use This Supplement for . . .

- A youth who continues to struggle with anhedonia (things are not as much fun as they used to be).
- A youth who withdrew from activities throughout the course of depression and is having a difficult time getting involved in activities again.
- A youth who frequently complains (either in therapy or to parents) of feeling bored.

SKILLS TO CONSIDER

- Behavioral coping
- Cognitive restructuring and automatic thoughts

STRATEGIES TO TRY

1. Behavioral coping: Look back at Handout 6.7, Behavioral Coping Skills (any activities listed as Distracting and Fun, Relaxing and Soothing, Expend Energy, Something Social, Something that makes you feel successful). Consider adding an activity to this list.

2. If the youth was not able to think of any activities that are enjoyable currently, reference the timeline: Were there any activities that the youth did before he or she was depressed? What would the youth be doing if he were not "bored"? How does the youth want to make the timeline look in the future regarding activities?

3. Behavioral coping activity in the office: If the youth is having trouble generating enjoyable activities at home, it could be helpful to do a behavioral coping activity during the session (e.g., hula-hoop, office ballgame, going on a walk). Ask the youth to rate his or her mood before and after the activity.

4. Behavioral coping and problem solving: activity scheduling. In the session, help the youth to plan a time during the next week to engage in certain activities. Generate possible barriers to completing the activities and problem-solve (Curry et al., 2000).

   - Use a weekly schedule or log and plan for activities either hourly or by periods/ chunks of the day. Work with the youth to fill in the schedule and contract with the youth to complete these activities. Make the activities specific.

   - If the youth is willing, consider having him or her rate either the mood after each activity or possibly his or her mastery of or pleasure for each activity. You may use Handout 6.2, Mood Thermometer, as a guide (look for both pleasure and success).

- Problem-solve barriers to task completion. Use the parents for support.

5. Cognitive restructuring: Review automatic negative thoughts. Work with the youth to generate a list of automatic negative thoughts that may contribute to the anhedonia. Start the youth off with statements such as: "This is so dumb," "I can't believe I am doing this," "I never have fun . . . (playing soccer, at the movies, going over to someone's house)."

- Look at the activities that the youth is currently trying or has been involved with in the past.
- Elicit the youth's evaluations of these activities.
- Explore the possibility that the youth's automatic negative thoughts are getting in the way of enjoying these activities.
- Relate being bored/uninterested in activities to being "stuck" in a bad mood. Refer to the car metaphor used on page 56 in Session 2 (anhedonia is kind of like pulling over and stopping—it's hard to get back in the flow of traffic once you've pulled over).
- Work with the youth to generate realistic counterthoughts that could help him or her to get "unstuck" or out of the boredom. Examples: "I remember when this used to be fun and really believe that it could be fun again," "This is more fun than . . . (taking a test, cleaning my room)," "This could be fun if I just give it a chance."

6. Apply to the timeline: Discuss activities that the youth was involved in prior to feeling depressed. Discuss the importance of having enjoyable activities as part of your relapse prevention plan. Talk about the effect of inactivity on mood and how increasing activities and ways to enjoy yourself can increase mood. Talk about the lethargy and lack of motivation that come with depression and how staying active and involved can be part of the Wellness Plan.

SUGGESTED HANDOUTS

✓ Behavioral Coping Skills (Handout 6.7)

✓ Activity Scheduling (Handout 6.8)

Boredom Supplement

Use This Supplement for . . .

- A youth who continues to struggle with anhedonia (things are not as much fun as they used to be).
- A youth who withdrew from activities throughout the course of depression and is having a difficult time getting involved in activities again.
- A youth who frequently complains (either in therapy or to parents) of feeling bored.

SKILLS TO CONSIDER

- Behavioral coping
- Cognitive restructuring and automatic thoughts
- Problem solving

STRATEGIES TO TRY

1. Behavioral coping: Look at Handout 6.7, Behavioral Coping Skills (any activities listed as Distracting and Fun, Relaxing and Soothing, Expend Energy, Something Social, Something that makes you feel successful). Consider adding an activity to this list.

2. If the youth was not able to think of any activities that were enjoyable currently, reference the timeline. Were there any activities that the youth did before he or she was depressed? What would the youth be doing if he or she were not "bored"? How does the youth want to make the timeline regarding activities look in the future?

3. Behavioral coping and problem solving: Look at Handout 6.8, Activity Scheduling. In the session, help the youth to plan a time during the next week to engage in certain activities. Generate possible barriers to completing the activities and problem-solve ways to manage obstacles.

   - Use a weekly schedule or log and plan for activities either hourly or by periods or chunks of the day. Work with the youth to fill in the schedule and contract with the youth to complete these activities. Make the activities specific.

   - If the youth is willing, consider having him or her rate either his or her mood after each activity or possibly his or her mastery or pleasure for each activity. A mood rating scale can be used as a guide. Look for both pleasure and success.

   - Problem-solve barriers to task completion.

4. Cognitive restructuring: Review automatic negative thoughts. Work with the youth to generate a list of automatic negative thoughts that may contribute to the experience of boredom. Start the youth off with statements like: "This is so dumb," "I can't believe I am doing this," "This is the stupidest thing ever," "I never have fun (playing soccer, at the movies, going over to someone's house)."

- Look at the activities that youth is currently trying or has been involved with in the past.

- Elicit the youth's evaluations of these activities.

- Explore the possibility that the youth's automatic negative thoughts are getting in the way of enjoying these activities.

- Relate being bored to being "stuck" in a bad mood. Refer again to the car metaphor (boredom can be kind of like pulling over and stopping—it's hard to get back in the flow of traffic once you've pulled over).

- Work with the youth to generate realistic counterthoughts that could help him or her to get "unstuck" or out of the boredom. Examples: "I remember when this used to be fun and really believe that it could be fun again," "This is more fun than (taking a test, cleaning my room)," "This could be fun if I just give it a chance."

5. Problem solving. Use FLIP with specific situations in which the youth has felt bored. Consider using vignettes to apply problem-solving techniques.

6. Apply to the timeline: Discuss activities that the youth was involved in before feeling depressed. Discuss the importance of having enjoyable activities as part of a lapse prevention plan. Talk about the effect of boredom on mood and how increasing activities can improve mood. Talk about the lethargy and lack of motivation that come with depression and how staying active and involved can be part of the wellness plan.

SUGGESTED HANDOUTS

✓ Behavioral Coping Skills (Handout 6.7)

✓ Activity Scheduling (Handout 6.8)

Emotion Regulation Supplement

Use This Supplement for . . .

- A youth who reports residual difficulties managing emotions or for whom emotional regulation was difficult when depressed.

- A youth who has a more irritable depression; consider using emotion regulation as the primary focus of one or more sessions.

- Application to any intense emotion that puts the youth at risk for relapse and/or causes problems for the youth, including anger and anxiety.

SKILLS TO CONSIDER

- Automatic negative thoughts and cognitive restructuring
- Behavioral coping

STRATEGIES TO TRY

1. Create a personalized Mood Thermometer to increase the youth's awareness of his or her intense emotions and to teach the youth that emotions exist on a continuum, rather than being "all-or-nothing." Teach the youth to identify when he or she is at risk for losing control of intense emotions.

   - Identify anchors:

     ○ Calmest point = 0: *"In what kind of situation are you a 0?"; "When is the last time that you remember feeling completely calm?"*

     ○ "Boiling" or "out of control" point = 10: *"In what kind of situation are you a 10?"; "When is the last time that you remember feeling completely out of control?"; "When was the last time that you lost control?"*

     ○ Fill in the range between the two emotions: "Hot zone" is the range leading up to the "boiling point," the range in which the youth is at risk of losing control of his or her emotions or "boiling over."

     ○ The youth should identify the point where he or she is about to lose control, right below the boiling point but still in the hot zone. This is the point where the emotion is very strong (intense), but the youth is still able to control his or her behaviors.

   - Identify the behavioral cues (e.g., pacing, hitting hand, clenching your fist, raising your voice, crying), cognitive cues (e.g., "I can't stand this," "I want to get out of here," "I want to hit someone"), and physiological cues (e.g., heart pounding, feeling hot, sweating, red in the face, stomachache, tension, feeling tingly or numb) that signal when the youth is in the hot zone.

2. Teach the youth to use realistic counterthoughts and/or cognitive restructuring to modify automatic negative thoughts when in the hot zone.

3. Teach the youth to use behavioral coping skills and/or self-soothing when he or she catches himself or herself in the hot zone to distract from or cope with the situation.

4. Discuss with the youth past situations in which he or she has been prone to emotional disregulation. Work with the youth to anticipate future situations in which he or she is at risk for emotional disregulation. Work with the youth to contrast how the "Old" Me would handle a stressful situation versus how the "Best" Me, equipped with several new skills, would handle it.

> **THERAPIST TIP:** It is important that the youth practice strategies for emotional regulation when he or she is *not* in a stressful situation. The youth will be better equipped to access his or her strategies for emotional regulation if he or she has practiced or "rehearsed" using them. Some youth find that using index cards and putting the information in their phones are helpful reminders of specific strategies to use when they find themselves in the hot zone.

SUGGESTED HANDOUTS

✓ Mood Thermometer (Handout 6.2)

✓ The "Best" Me (Handout 11.3)

Hopelessness Supplement

Use This Supplement for . . .

- A youth who expresses hopelessness about his or her future, in general, or about further improvement of his or her depressive symptoms.

> **THERAPIST TIP:** Hopelessness has been linked to relapse in adolescents (Brent et al., 1999). Making this connection and understanding the rationale for combating hopelessness are important components of the intervention.

SKILLS TO CONSIDER

- Cognitive restructuring and automatic thoughts

STRATEGIES TO TRY

1. Introduce the idea of hopelessness, the continuum of hopelessness, and the relationship of hopelessness to mood. Just as changing thoughts changes mood, we can use thoughts to change feelings of hopelessness.

2. Cognitive restructuring: Work with the youth to identify the negative automatic thoughts that might be contributing to the feeling of hopelessness (e.g., "Nothing ever works out for me," "There's no use in trying") and then restructure the cognitions in a way that instills hope (e.g., "I'm frustrated right now, but I'm going to try because some things do work out for me").

3. Cognitive restructuring: Conceptualization of a continuum with "hopelessness" on one end and "hopefulness" at the other end. In an early session, assess the youth's level of hopelessness by asking him or her to mark an "X" corresponding to where on the continuum he or she falls at that time. At future sessions, reassess the youth's level of hopelessness using a fresh continuum worksheet. If the youth's level of hopelessness has improved (even if by only a small degree) from a prior hopelessness assessment, pull out the previously used continuum and compare it to the current one. This comparison can serve as evidence that feelings of hopelessness fluctuate in a way similar to mood (e.g., "Just because I feel hopeless now does not mean that I will always feel hopeless") and thus can be a powerful intervention.

4. Cognitive restructuring: Use the hopefulness pie chart. Have the youth plot his or her degree of hopefulness on a pie chart. What ingredients can we put in the pie to increase the size of the 'hopeful' slice of the pie (i.e., hopefulness operationalized; "What would you be doing/thinking if you were more hopeful?")?

5. Problem solving: Reasons to be hopeful. Once the youth can look at the concept of hopelessness on a continuum, it is important to talk with the youth about things that make him or her more hopeful about life and about treatment. During this discussion, collaborate to generate the youth's reasons for hope. Explore with the youth things he or she looks forward to. How can he or she increase the number of things to look forward to? Depressed mood and/or feelings of irritability impair our ability to recall our reasons for hope. (Relate to the youth's timeline, "Have you had a time in the past when you felt so low that you had a hard time remembering the positive things in your life?") Make the connection between "hope" and "control": "Hope" is something that is changeable and therefore something the youth can control.

THERAPIST TIP: Tie hopefulness and hopelessness to the timeline. Similarly, comparisons can be made between the current level of hopelessness and the youth's level of hopelessness when he or she was depressed using the timeline.

SUGGESTED HANDOUT

✓ Continuum of Hope (Handout A.3)

Impulsivity Supplement

Use This Supplement for . . .

* A youth who has difficulty with impulsive and/or deviant behavior

SKILLS TO CONSIDER

* Emotional regulation
* Problem solving

STRATEGIES TO TRY

1. Emotional regulation, behavioral coping, and cognitive restructuring: Work with the youth to complete the mood thermometer in the Emotional Regulation supplement. Many adolescents will report that their behavior occurs so quickly that they don't have a chance to think about it. Ask the youth to give a specific example of impulsive behavior and then to describe the situation. Identify the specific physiological, psychological, and behavioral cues that suggest that the youth is about to act impulsively. Using these cues, create a list of warning signs or "red flags" that can alert the youth that he or she is in danger of acting impulsively. The goal is to help the youth recognize the urge to act before the behavior occurs. Use the youth's language to describe these urges and the signals that he or she is getting close to acting without thinking through the consequences. Then, the youth can use behavioral coping and/or cognitive restructuring strategies to calm himself or herself down and to resist the urge.

2. *Decision-check* is a specific strategy to help a youth overcome an action urge. Its rationale is that if the youth stops to evaluate the possible negative consequences of an action urge, the likelihood of resisting that urge improves. The youth should be socialized to the strategy language, such as the decision-check phase, which should trigger the youth to think about the consequences before succumbing to an action urge. The reminder to conduct a decision-check could come from a friend or family member who verbally reminds the youth to conduct a decision-check. Conversely, it could be in the form of strategically placed note cards (with decision-check written on them).

   * For example, a youth who has the action urge to sneak out of his or her house at night might post a decision-check card on his or her bedroom window. Similarly, a younger youth who impulsively gets out of his or her seat in the classroom might post a decision-check card on his or her desk or notebook.

- It should be noted that the patient might wish to use a different phrase to trigger an evaluation of consequences (e.g., "STOP," "Is it worth it?"). This should be encouraged. You can adopt the youth's exact language when working on this skill with that youth.

3. Problem solving: Identify risk factors or high-risk situations for impulsivity. Problem-solve (FLIP) ways to add in a delay or pause to allow the youth to weigh the consequences prior to engaging in the high-risk behavior.

  - For example, if a friend who often asks the youth to engage in high-risk activities calls the youth to go out, the youth should attempt to "buy himself or herself time" by saying, "I need to check my calendar and get back to you."

SUGGESTED HANDOUTS

✓ FLIP the Problem (Handout 8.1)

Interpersonal Conflict Supplement

Use This Supplement for . . .

- A youth who has difficulty with negotiation, feeling that he or she never gets what he or she wants.

- A youth who has difficulty compromising in family, social, and academic settings.

- A family that has difficulty with problem solving and communication.

SKILLS TO CONSIDER

- Assertiveness supplement
- Social skills development supplement
- Cognitive restructuring and automatic thoughts
- Problem solving

STRATEGIES TO TRY

1. Cognitive restructuring.

   - Explore recent situations involving interpersonal conflict, identify the youth's role in the conflict, and look for skills that may be needed (check the above supplements). Identify the automatic negative thoughts and cognitive distortions that contribute to the conflict. Difficulties in compromising can be related to automatic thoughts or cognitive distortions.

   - Using examples from the role plays or examples the youth has brought up earlier in treatment, you may identify automatic thoughts or distortions that may get in the way of listening or of compromising.

2. Problem solving: Teach "social problem solving" using WIN from the Assertiveness Skill Supplement.

   - **W:** Wait and listen to what the other person is saying.
   - **I:** Use "I" statements to get what you want.
   - **N:** Negotiate a compromise to get what you want.
   - Apply WIN to different situations, preferably those from the youth's experience (use movie clips or vignettes if needed).

3. Problem solving: Introduce compromise as an extension of earlier problem-solving skills (FLIP). Key ideas to convey include:

- The need for compromise in any relationship.
- The relationship between compromise and problem solving.
- The connection between negative automatic thoughts/cognitive distortions and difficulty compromising.

4. *In vivo* interaction in the session with the therapist. Role-play both with the youth as him-/herself and with the youth as the other person.

5. Relate the social problem-solving skills covered in this supplement to earlier situations, incidents, or patterns brought up by the youth that suggest that inability to compromise is costing the youth social support or increasing family discord, peer conflict, or difficulty with teachers—all of which can contribute to depression.

6. Introduce the idea of "give and take" to the youth.

7. Relate this skill to the timeline. Introduce ways that this skill will be useful in the future, such as in college with roommates or in a dating situation.

SUGGESTED HANDOUTS

✓ WIN (Handout A.2)

✓ FLIP the Problem (Handout 8.1)

Irritability Supplement

Use This Supplement for . . .

- A youth who reports a feeling of being "on edge" or easily angered.
- A youth who has difficulty getting along with friends and parents or says that everyone is "getting on my nerves."
- A youth who seems surly or uncooperative in sessions.

> **THERAPIST TIP:** Irritability has been found to be a common residual symptom in adults (Fava et al., 1999), thus making this an especially important supplement.

SKILLS TO CONSIDER

- Family expressed emotion (from behavioral coping session)
- Cognitive restructuring and automatic thoughts
- Problem solving
- Social skills supplement
- Emotion regulation supplement

STRATEGIES TO TRY

1. It is important to determine whether irritability is something that the youth experiences with individuals or in situations outside of the family. If irritability occurs exclusively within the family, the Family Expressed Emotion module in Session 2 should be revisited and further communication skills between parent and youth should be incorporated.

2. Cognitive restructuring: Irritability as related to mood. *"Do you seem to be more irritable when you are feeling sad?"*

3. Behavioral coping and problem solving: What other factors contribute to irritability for you? Suggested factors to consider:
   - Lack of sleep
   - Hunger
   - Stress
   - Lack of exercise

- Overwhelmed with school due to missed work, procrastination, or excessive demands
- Sarcasm: using or receiving

4. Cognitive restructuring.
- Discuss the irritability in the context of a mood monitor. Use a Mood Monitor to get details regarding irritability such as, when is it more likely to occur, in what situations, and with whom? Once situations or relationships have been identified as "at risk for irritability," explore automatic negative thoughts.
- Explain the rationale for using this skill.

  "When you have automatic negative thoughts that are related to how you feel about yourself, these thoughts can really bring your mood down and make you feel sad or bad about yourself. Automatic negative thoughts can also bring your mood down and anger and irritability up when you have them about other people."

5. Cognitive restructuring: Generate a list of automatic negative thoughts about others and/or situations encountered frequently that result in irritability. Look for alternative attributions or more helpful ways to think about others:
- Be sure to include all of the people that the youth perceives as irritating (e.g., parents, teachers, friends, siblings, the therapist).
- Examples: "He is so stupid"; "They are trying to get me in trouble"; "They will never understand me"; "I can't believe she would ask such a dumb question."
- Explore angry statements and be aware of cognitive distortions.
- Choose a situation in which the youth was irritable. Avoid "hot" issues such as conflict with parents. Lower intensity issues are more conducive to teaching and applying skills. Have the youth describe the situation in detail. As the youth is describing the situation, say some of the negative thoughts from the youth's list out loud. Demonstrate how these thoughts can "fan the flames" and increase irritability. When the youth seems to be more irritated with the situation, ask the youth to rate his or her mood.
- Ask the youth to discuss the same situation again. This time, model realistic counter thoughts.
- Ask the youth to rate his or her mood. Link thoughts with mood and behaviors.

> **SUGGESTED HANDOUT**
> ✓ Irritability (Handout A.4)

Peer Victimization (Dealing with Bullies) Supplement

Use This Supplement for . . .

- A youth who feels alienated as a result of ridicule, teasing, or rejection from peers.

SKILLS TO CONSIDER

- Social skills supplement
- Social support supplement
- Assertiveness supplement
- Problem solving

STRATEGIES TO TRY

1. Problem solving: Ask the youth what he or she has already done to prevent/cope with the bullying. Evaluate whether or not the strategy was effective. Identify the positive strategies that the youth uses and bring them to the youth's attention.

2. Problem solving: Identify precipitants that lead to conflict such as verbal and nonverbal communication, as well as specific situations where the youth is more at risk for being bullied. It is important for the youth to be aware of factors that contribute to the bullying and the role that he or she plays in the situation. Brainstorm possible methods of communication that welcome bullying behavior, both nonverbal (nose picking, hot face, crossing arms, crying) and verbal (hostile remarks to provoke the bully).

3. Problem solving: Use a recent example of bullying and apply the problem-solving method (FLIP) to teach the youth how to deal with future bullying situations.

   - **F:** Figure out what the problem is and what you want.
   - **L:** List all possible solutions. Collaborate with the youth to explore the possibilities. Possible examples are:
     - Escape or avoid situations where the bullying occurs.
     - Have the youth fight back in an appropriate manner such as acting assertively.
     - The youth could act cool as if the teasing doesn't bother him or her.
     - The youth could seek help from teachers, parents, or friends.
   - **I:** Identify the best solution.
   - **P:** Plan when and where to use this strategy. Then assess the outcome of using the strategy.

4. Behavioral coping: To cope with bullying, explore and expand the social network. Consider using a supplement on social skills or social support.

5. Behavioral coping: Role-play a personal situation of bullying that occurs. Ask the youth to alternate playing both the role of the bully and the victim. What did the youth learn in his or her role-playing experience?

6. Problem solving: Have the youth predict the next time a bullying situation is likely to occur. Help the youth to create a plan of how to cope with the situation using the FLIP method.

7. Problem solving: For a younger youth, review how to seek help and identify whom to ask for help.

8. Cognitive restructuring: For a more cognitive youth, identify the locus of control and feelings of helplessness.

SUGGESTED HANDOUTS

✓ FLIP the Problem (Handout 8.1)

✓ Social Situation Tracker (Handout A.5)

Relaxation Training and Sleep Hygiene Supplement

Use This Supplement for . . .

- A youth who has difficulty with relaxation, anxiety, or tension.
- A youth who has sleep problems.

SKILLS TO CONSIDER

- Cognitive restructuring and automatic thoughts
- Emotional regulation

STRATEGIES TO TRY

1. Basic relaxation techniques: These techniques form the foundation of relaxation. For each of the following strategies, model the techniques for the youth and then have the youth practice in the session, as appropriate.
   - Deep breathing
     - Hold hand over your belly and breathe deeply so that your hand can feel each breath. Your belly will expand as you breathe in and retract as you breathe out.
     - Pretend that you are blowing a bubble as you breathe out.
     - Suggest breathing through the mouth.
   - Muscle relaxation
     - Practice clenching fists and relaxing.
     - Clench feet and relax.
     - Suck in stomach and relax.
     - You can practice a muscle relaxation on any part of your body. The ones included here are easy to do in public places (school, social situations).
   - Positive self-statements
     - Identify the automatic negative thought(s) that may be contributing to tension and anxiety.
     - Use counterthoughts and positive self-statements to "talk back to" automatic negative thoughts that may be fostering tension.
     - Examples: "I am feeling more relaxed each minute," "I can feel my muscles relaxing."

2. If tension is a more significant issue and more intervention is needed, consider the following techniques:
  - Progressive muscle relaxation through more of the body
    - Start at the toes: Clench and release.
    - Legs: Clench and release.
    - Shoulders: Clench and release.
    - Torso/stomach: Clench and release.
    - Talk the youth through major, large muscle groups.
  - Deep breathing with self-statements
    - As you breathe in, say "I am gathering up all of the tension in my body."
    - As you breathe out, say "I am letting all of the tension go."
  - Deep breathing with pleasant imagery
    - Brainstorm a list of places that the youth finds most relaxing.
    - Ask the youth to describe these places in detail, appealing to as many senses as possible. For example, if the youth finds the beach to be relaxing, have him or her think of how the sun feels on the back, how the sand feels between the toes, what the ocean smells like, the sound of the ocean waves, and so on.
    - As the youth breathes in and out, have him or her close his or her eyes and focus on one aspect of the relaxing place.

3. If tension is a primary focus of the youth's presentation and more intervention is needed:
  - Progressive muscle relaxation—throughout the body
    - Direct the youth to tense and relax each part of the body beginning with the toes and ending with the shoulders.
    - Work with the youth to make a tape recording of self-soothing/coaching statements to guide progressive muscle relaxation.
  - Deep breathing with self-statements and counting backward (adapted from Curry et al., 2000)
    - Have the youth practice counting backward with each deep breath.
    - After the youth has counted from 10 back to 8, introduce self-statements: "I feel more relaxed at 7 than I did at 8" and so on."
    - Identify the self-statements that accompany each gradation of relaxation. Make the link from thoughts to mood/relaxation.
  - Guided imagery
    - See Koeppen (1974) for the full reference.

4. Review the youth's recent sleep schedule and sleep hygiene practices. Explore with the youth any issues that might be affecting his or her sleep, such as staying up late using the computer, watching TV late at night, or using caffeine. Review Handout A.6, Well Rested: Tips for Better Sleep, and collaborate with the youth to create a plan for improved sleep.

SUGGESTED HANDOUTS

✓ Behavioral Coping Skills (Handout 6.7)

✓ Well Rested: Tips for Better Sleep (Handout A.6)

✓ Sleep Log (Handout A.7)

Self-Esteem Supplement

Use This Supplement for . . .

* A youth who feels inferior or unworthy, values others more than the self, or has trouble recognizing his or her own strengths.

SKILLS TO CONSIDER

* Emotion regulation supplement
* Assertiveness supplement
* Cognitive restructuring and automatic thoughts

STRATEGIES TO TRY

1. Tie self-esteem into the timeline. Ask the youth what positive self-esteem means to him or her? How would he or she rate his or her self-esteem? How does he or she think positive self-esteem would have been helpful in the past and now in the present? How will having positive self-esteem affect the youth in the future (e.g., have more friends, be more outgoing, not worry about what other people think)?

> **THERAPIST TIP:** The youth may need to have the term *self-esteem* defined.
>
> *"Self-esteem refers to how you think and feel about yourself. Sometimes we have trouble recognizing our strengths and accepting the positive things that we are capable of doing. Positive self-esteem is important to maintain wellness and prevent relapse."*

2. Cognitive restructuring: Identify the positive. Ask the youth to identify and list positive characteristics about himself or herself. What are the things that he or she does well? What are common compliments that the youth receives? Identify the different roles that the youth plays, such as son, daughter, student, brother, sister, and friend. What would people say about him or her in these roles?

3. Cognitive restructuring: Identify negative thoughts. Help the youth to identify negative thoughts by discussing a situation that went poorly for the youth or asking the youth to list things that he or she is not good at. Use Handout A.8, Self-Esteem Check, to identify the youth's negative automatic thoughts. Teach the youth to challenge the negative messages. Normalize that many youths with low self-esteem have a critical inner voice, but that it is important to be able to challenge those thoughts. Identify thinking errors used by the youth. Could the youth be minimizing the positive?

4. Build a positive self-schema.

- Behavioral coping: Ask the youth to identify what he or she thinks are his or her positive qualities. What are the activities that the youth enjoys? How does the youth feel when he or she is engaging in an activity that he or she enjoys? Incorporate the behavioral coping skill.

- Cognitive restructuring: Make a list of positive self-statements. How could these be practiced and incorporated into the homework?

5. Body language: Operationalize high self-esteem and the behavioral manifestations of strong self-esteem. Discuss with the youth what having positive self-esteem would look like.

- For example, sitting up straight, making eye contact, and smiling are examples of behavioral manifestations of strong self-esteem.

- When the youth uses this body language, ask how it makes him or her feel? What would the youth be doing differently if he or she had more self-esteem or thought more of himself or herself?

- Cognitive restructuring: Ask the youth to identify the cognitive manifestations of high self-esteem. What thoughts are associated with positive views of self? What would the youth be saying to himself or herself if he or she had high self-esteem?

SUGGESTED HANDOUT

✓ Self-Esteem Check (Handout A.8)

Social Skills Supplement

Use This Supplement for . . .

- A youth who does not interact socially because he or she lacks basic skills in peer relatedness.

- A youth who has difficulty with social cues, socially appropriate behavior, and social interactions.

SKILLS TO CONSIDER

- Automatic negative thoughts and cognitive restructuring

STRATEGIES TO TRY

1. Focus on the role of cognition in the youth's difficulty with social interactions. Teach the youth that what we say to ourselves before we interact with others can influence the outcome of the interaction. Recognizing your thoughts about your ability to relate to others is the key to making things go better socially.

   "For example, if you say 'No one is going to ask me to sit with them at lunch. No one notices me, I am invisible,' what do you think these thoughts would lead to? Do you think they would increase your likelihood of talking to someone, or if they would decrease your likelihood? What would you do if you had these thoughts?"

   - Remind the youth of the triangle, and highlight the relationships of thoughts and behaviors.

   - Work with the youth to identify negative automatic thoughts and then replace those thoughts with restructured thoughts that might improve the outcome of the social situation. If the youth has difficulty identifying negative automatic thoughts, work with the youth to develop a list of positive self-statements that promote positive social behavior.

   THERAPIST TIP: Look for thoughts that relate to self-schemas, such as "I am unlikable" or "I am not popular."

2. Help the youth to recognize these basic ingredients for a positive social interaction:

   - Having positive thoughts about your ability to engage with the other person.

   - Predicting success in the interaction.

- Making eye contact.
- Smiling.
- Showing reciprocity of conversation.
- Making on-topic comments.
- Having an opening line.
- Thinking of a good topic.
- Making a positive comment about the other person.

3. Help the youth to become aware of patterns during his or her week when interaction with others is necessary or unnecessary. Using the Social Situation Tracker, Handout A.5, go through a typical week with the youth, identifying particularly awkward times (e.g., lunch time, soccer games on Saturday, Friday night football games) and particularly successful times (e.g., in a marching band with other clarinet players, one on one with a friend from church). Help the youth identify the specific cues around these positive and negative situations.

4. Consider these routine social situations to review and practice:
- Starting a conversation.
- Breaking into a group conversation.
- Having listening skills.
- Ending a one-on-one conversation.
- Leaving a group conversation.

These can be role-played with the youth, using Handout A.9, Small Talk Tips, as a guide. Consider role-playing the "right way" and the "wrong way" to respond to a particular situation. Point out the strengths of the youth's role play, as well as areas for improvements.

SUGGESTED HANDOUTS

✓ Small Talk Tips (Handout A.9)

✓ Social Situation Tracker (Handout A.5)

Social Support Supplement

Use This Supplement for . . .

- A youth who needs to increase his or her social network.
- A youth who has difficulty choosing friends who have a positive effect on his or her life.

SKILLS TO CONSIDER

- Problem solving
- Wellness

STRATEGIES TO TRY

1. If necessary, provide a rationale for developing/strengthening social support.

   "Social support or having good relationships with friends is an important part of preventing relapse. Having good friends (friends who bring your mood up) will improve mood, promote wellness, and decrease the risk of the depression coming back. Social support can help insulate you from relapse, so this is a good time to evaluate the friendships that you already have, as well as to make new friends."

2. Teach the youth about the influence of friends and how to assess relationships.

   - Using Handout 5.1, Self-Triangle, demonstrate the influence of friends on our thoughts, feelings, and behaviors (cognitive triad). Reference the behavioral coping and wellness skills to stress that social relationships are an important and necessary part of life.

   - Assess the youth's relationships, using the timeline, in the past (before depression and during depression) and in the present. What was the status of friendships? How are the friendships now? How would the youth like them to be? "In the past, what symptoms of your depression made it difficult for you to be around your friends?" If applicable, introduce the idea of "sand bags" (using the metaphor of the hot air balloon). "Sand bags are behaviors that some of your friends might engage in that bring you down. These may include alcohol and drug use and antisocial behavior."

3. Introduce the idea that different friends meet different needs for the youth. It is not wise to invest all of your time and emotional energy in just one friendship (i.e., put "all of your eggs in one basket"). Bring in Handout 9.2, Who's on Your

Team?, and complete it with the youth. Identify people the youth goes to for support or problems, those he or she goes to for fun, and so on.

> **THERAPIST TIP:** Identify social goals, current assets/strengths to increase, as well as targets for intervention. For example, if depression made the youth withdraw from activities, then this needs to be emphasized. Focus on the areas that the youth needs help with (i.e., activity involvement, choice of friends, social isolation, social obstacles).

4. Teach the youth to MAKE good choices about friendships.

- **M:** Match yourself with people who have similar interests, goals, or lifestyles.

    "When making new friends or evaluating old friendships, it is important to think about the people that you are wanting to spend your time with. What does this person like to do? What do you like to do? What are similar hobbies that you both have? What hobbies do you have that are not alike? Is school important to this person? Is family important? Is having a boyfriend or girlfriend important? Are these things important to you?

    "It is not necessary to only spend time with people who are exactly like you—differences are what make people interesting! But it is important that your friends share your views on any issues that are really important to you. For example, if getting good grades is really important to you, because of your long-term goals, then it probably would not be a good idea for you to spend a lot of time with someone who encourages you to study less, thus negatively affecting your goals. It would still be possible to be friends with this person, but you probably would want to limit your contact with him or her."

- **A:** Actively seek out relationships that are positive.

    "It is a good idea to make an effort to spend more time with those individuals who make you feel happy or satisfied. On the other hand, you should probably minimize your time with friends who lead you to feel more depressed, bored, or dissatisfied."

- **K:** Know how friends affect your mood and behaviors.

    "Remember that friends impact your thoughts, feelings, and behaviors (cognitive triad). In turn, your thoughts, feelings, and behaviors affect your well-being and mood. Since the goal of this treatment is to avoid a relapse into depression, it is important to keep in mind the potential mood busters that exist and to take steps to avoid these things."

- **E:** Evaluate your mood when with your friends.

"Remember to monitor your mood when spending time with your friends. Pay attention to your mood thermometer before spending time with a friend, and compare the rating to how you feel after spending time with a friend. To prevent depression, it may be a good idea to spend most of your time with friends who improve your mood rating, versus those who make your mood rating go down."

SUGGESTED HANDOUTS

✓ Lift Your Mood (Handout 6.9)

✓ Who's on Your Team? (Handout 9.2)

✓ MAKE (Handout A.10)

Suicidality: Guidelines for Management

THERAPIST TIP: The appropriateness of this relapse prevention treatment should be evaluated by the therapist and a supervisor when a youth expresses high or frequent suicidal ideation and/or behavior.

1. Assess the intent, severity, frequency, and duration of suicidal thoughts and/or behaviors.
   a. Decision point: Is outpatient treatment appropriate based on the level of severity? If Yes, continue.
   b. If No, consider referral options.
2. Create a safety plan.
   a. Secure an agreement from the youth to follow the safety plan (i.e., to promise to be safe and to follow the plan until the next session).
   b. Create a plan with specific steps and coping behaviors to prevent acting on suicidal thoughts or urges. Also include emergency contact numbers and crisis procedures in the safety plan.
   c. Secure the environment (no access to pills, knives, guns, ropes, etc.).
   d. Involve the parents in the plan. Contract with the parents to table issues that are causing conflict and upheaval ("hot topics") until suicidality (behaviors and thoughts) subsides; parents need to keep the environment safe.
3. Identify skills to reduce depressed mood and manage suicidality.
4. Evaluate and monitor the ideation closely.
   a. Make sure that the level of supervision is appropriate.
   b. Track outcomes.

ADDITIONAL SUPPLEMENTS AND SKILLS

- Emotion Regulation Supplement
- Hopelessness Supplement
- Cognitive restructuring and automatic thoughts

ADDITIONAL REFERENCES

- National Suicide Prevention Lifeline Safety Plan (*www.suicidepreventionlifeline.org/learn/safety.aspx*)
- Suicide Prevention Resource Center (*www.sprc.org*) has safety plan templates (*www.sprc.org/sites/sprc.org/files/SafetyPlanTemplate.pdf*)

BREAK

Take a

B: Believe in coping skill.

R: Relaxation techniques.

E: Evaluate the situation.

A: Alarm—false or real?

K: Keep your cool.

WIN

BE ASSERTIVE &

BE ASSERTIVE & . . .

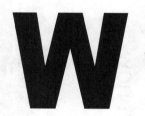

Wait and listen to what the other person is saying.

Use **"I"** statements.

Negotiate a compromise to get what you want.

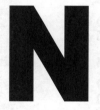

When would you like to be assertive?

_____

_____

What stops you from being assertive?

_____

_____

CONTINUUM OF HOPE

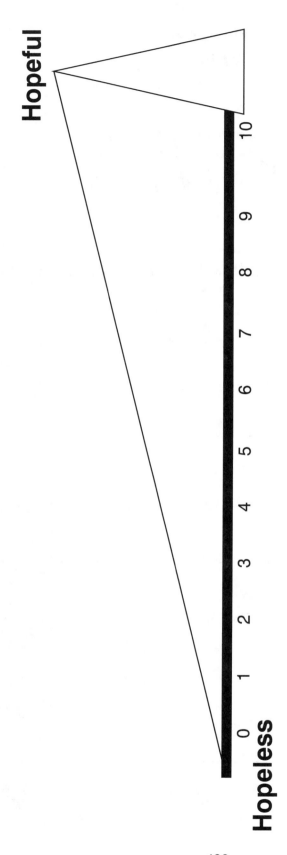

Hopeful

Hopeless

0 1 2 3 4 5 6 7 8 9 10

How hopeful do you feel right now?

IRRITABILITY

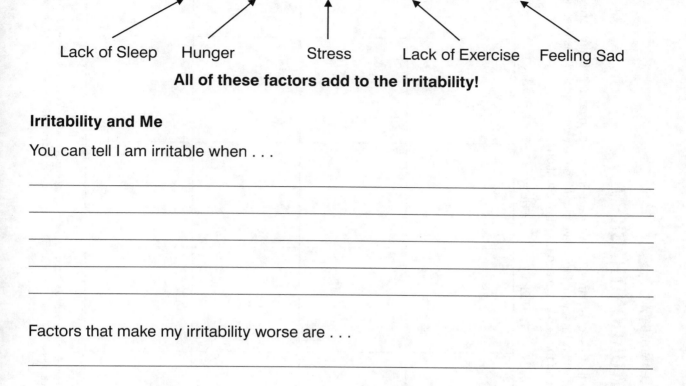

Lack of Sleep   Hunger   Stress   Lack of Exercise   Feeling Sad

All of these factors add to the irritability!

Irritability and Me

You can tell I am irritable when . . .

_____

_____

_____

_____

_____

Factors that make my irritability worse are . . .

_____

_____

_____

_____

Ways to prevent my irritability are . . .

_____

_____

_____

_____

_____

SOCIAL SITUATION TRACKER

Complete this worksheet to show day-to-day social situations that are often stressful/awkward or good/enjoyable. Identify particularly stressful or awkward times during the week. Indicate social situations that you participate in during the week that are positive. How do these situations make you feel? Identify the specific cues around these positive and negative situations.

	Monday	Tuesday	Wednesday	Thursday	Friday	Saturday	Sunday
Morning							
Afternoon							
Evening							
Night							

WELL RESTED: TIPS FOR BETTER SLEEP

Watch fluids—Too many fluids before bedtime may cause you to wake up in the middle of the night.

Electronics—Electronics (including computers and cell phones) should be put away or turned off before bedtime.

Lessen naps—While naps can be tempting when you're tired, try to avoid them.

Limit time spent in bed—If you cannot fall asleep, do not lie in bed past 15–20 minutes. Get up and do a quiet activity. Avoid watching TV or going into a well-lit room, as this may wake you up further.

Relax—Try to do something soothing, like taking a hot bath or listening to relaxing music, before bedtime.

Exercise—Exercise is good for overall sleep, but make sure to do it long before bedtime. Do not exercise for 4–6 hours before bedtime.

Stop caffeine and alcohol—Stop drinking caffeine 4–6 hours prior to bedtime. Both caffeine and alcohol can have a negative impact on your sleep.

Train your brain—Your brain needs to learn that your bed is only for sleep. Avoid using it for other purposes such as doing homework, reading, or watching television.

Establish a bedtime and wake time—Do your bedtime and wake time vary? Your body gets used to patterns, and you can make this work for you by establishing a regular time for bed and waking.

Diet—Choosing the right foods can help your sleep! Large, spicy, or sugary meals before bedtime can cause difficultly in sleeping. Other foods, such as warm milk, chamomile tea, or bananas, may be good for sleep.

Adapted from the Treatment of Resistant Depression in Adolescents (TORDIA) study.

SLEEP LOG

	What time did you get into bed?	About how long did it take you to fall asleep?	What time did you wake up?	What time did you get out of bed?	Quality of sleep: Good Fair Poor	How many times did you wake up during the night?	If you had a nap, how long did you nap for?
Monday							
Tuesday							
Wednesday							
Thursday							
Friday							
Saturday							
Sunday							

Comments/Concerns

_____

_____

_____

_____

_____

SELF-ESTEEM CHECK

Check the boxes for the statements that are true for you. Discuss with the therapist the situations in which you felt this way. Add additional thoughts that you have about yourself at the bottom of the page.

☐ I am very sensitive.

☐ I am afraid that my friends think I am stupid.

☐ I am not comfortable experiencing new things.

☐ I try to hide my feelings from others.

☐ I try not to get close to anyone because I am afraid they will not like the real me.

☐ Everything is my fault.

☐ I am not as cute, funny, and smart as my friends.

☐ There are not that many good things to say about me.

☐ I don't have much to contribute to most conversations.

☐ All the good things that have happened to me are due to good luck.

☐ I have trouble accepting compliments from other people.

☐ I don't feel like I belong.

☐ I am scared of failure.

☐ I am always trying to please others and have trouble saying no.

☐ I sometimes feel lonely when others are around.

☐ I leave conversations worrying that I said the wrong thing.

☐ _____

SMALL TALK TIPS

Something you notice

- "You have the same backpack as me."

- "I have seen you on my school bus."

- _____

Something you like

- Give a compliment: "I like your shirt. Where did you get it?"

- "You did a good job on your presentation in class today."

- "Did you see _____ last night? It's my favorite show."

- _____

Something you know about

- "Have you seen any good movies? I just saw . . ."

- "I heard on the news . . ."

- _____

MAKE

M **M**atch yourself with people who have similar interests, goals, or lifestyles.

A **A**ctively seek out relationships that are positive.

K **K**now how friends affect your mood and behaviors.

E **E**valuate your mood when with your friends.

good choices about your

FRIENDSHIPS

Handouts for Parents

Introduction to Relapse Prevention CBT

Cognitive-Behavioral Model of Depression

- Three parts of the personality: emotions, thoughts, behaviors.
- Each part influences the other parts.

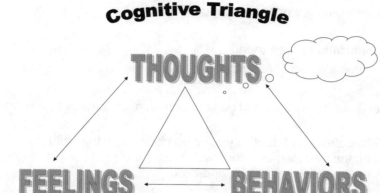

Relapse

- A "relapse" is the return of depression.
- Research shows that 30 to 40% of children and adolescents experience symptoms of depression again after completion of treatment.

Lapse versus Relapse

- It is expected that sometimes your child will have a "bad day" or be irritable or maybe even sad.
- A lapse (or brief return of a depressive symptom) DOES NOT EQUAL relapse.
- In this program, we will teach skills to help keep lapses from becoming a relapse.

Relapse Prevention CBT

- Certain skills are especially useful to help "fight depression" (i.e., decrease certain symptoms or problems).
- It is important to look back at the past events ("stressors") that may have contributed to depression in the child.
- It is also important to look at the present symptoms or problems that may be affecting the child's mood.

(continued)

Therapy Expectations

- The Four C's of Therapy: Collaboration, Communication, Confidentiality, Compliance
  - Collaboration
    - A team approach.
    - Sessions will include an agenda, which the child and therapist will create together.
    - Active homework, with an emphasis on thoughts/behaviors.
  - Communication
    - Two-way communication is important.
    - Feedback is appreciated and encouraged!
  - Confidentiality
    - The information kept by the child will be kept confidential; it will not be shared with parents/caretakers.
    - Limits of confidentiality: Confidentiality rules do not apply if the child is in danger or in any way unsafe. However, the therapist and child will discuss this in therapy and work together to come to a decision about what to say, when, and how.
  - Compliance
    - Each session will end with a homework or practice assignment, but this will be designed with the child.
    - Any obstacles to completing the homework will be addressed.
    - A challenge to any therapy program is the application of the skills outside of the session. Relapse prevention must be done daily, not just in sessions, for it to work.

Parental Involvement in Therapy

- The involvement of parents is important, as one of the best ways to prevent relapse is to have the proper support and reduce stress.
- A team approach can be helpful.
- Parents will be informed of skills (through handouts like this one), and the therapist will look for ways parents can help by reducing stress and conflict in the home and increasing support for the child.

Questions for the Therapist

- Use this space to write down any questions you may have for today:

Behavioral Coping Skills and Family Expressed Emotion

Mood = "Feelings"

- Understanding how you feel is the first step!
- Moods are not all good or bad, but vary along a continuum.
- Mood monitoring
  - A person can monitor his or her mood by thinking about the degrees on a thermometer, or the bars on a cell phone.
  - A scale of 1–10 is a way to rate mood and is a beginning step to be aware of mood changes or shifts.
  - What happens (thoughts/behaviors) to make the mood scale go up or down?

Mood Management

- Notice your mood patterns.
  - Changes during the day?
  - Relationships between behavior and mood?
  - Relationships between thoughts and mood?
- When your mood begins to go down, it is possible to stop and turn it around to avoid a "downward spiral."
  - When a stressor occurs, a person can let it continue to bring himself or herself down, letting the bad feelings gain momentum and spiral out of control . . . OR
  - When a stressor occurs, a person can work to change his or her mood.
- Ways to change mood
  - Two ways
    - Thinking
    - Doing
  - Today we will focus on "doing," which we call behavioral coping skills.

Behavioral Coping Skills

- Some people find that doing something can immediately help with their moods.
- We suggest:
  - Do something distracting and fun!
    - What activities do you enjoy?
    - What do you do "for fun"?
    - What makes you feel good?
    - How often do you do these activities?

(continued)

- Do something relaxing and soothing!
  - What makes you feel calm and relaxed?
    - A bubble bath?
    - A massage?
    - Reading?
    - Running?
  - How often do you do these things?
- Expend energy!
  - Physical activity has been shown to increase mood.
  - What do you do for exercise?
    - Run?
    - Play sports?
    - Rollerblade?
    - Dance?
  - How often do you do these things?
- Do something social!
  - Social support—getting help from others—is important to mood.
  - Social altruism—helping others—also improves mood!
  - What do you do with your friends?
  - What do you do to help others?
  - How often do you do these things?
- Do something that makes you feel successful!
  - We all like to succeed—it gives us a sense of mastery and improves self-esteem.
  - What are you good at?
  - What are you doing to improve your abilities in this area and others?
  - How often do you do these things?

Mood Busters!

- In contrast, certain activities and behaviors are guaranteed to bring you down and make you feel worse.
- What activities bring you down?
- How often do you do these things?
- How do these affect you?

(continued)

Today's Family Session

- Family Expressed Emotion
- Family "Temperature"
  - The communication and emotional level in a home can be thought of as being on a thermostat.
  - The "temperature" needs to be set at a level that is comfortable for all.
- Good Coach versus Bad Coach
  - A good coach is supportive of the player, even when mistakes are made.
  - Good behavior is praised, and bad behavior is corrected but with support and patience.
  - "Coaching style" can be a useful metaphor for parenting style.
- Negative Emotion at Home
  - It is common in families in which there are members with depression to have negative emotion: sarcasm, high levels of criticism, and low levels of positive reinforcement/praise.
  - Relapse in children and adolescents with depression occurs more frequently in families with high levels of negative emotion.
- Try to identify times when this occurs in your home.

Questions/Comments

- Have you thought of any other treatment goals for your child?
- How would you describe the "temperature" in your home? What is your coaching style?
- What can the family do to help the child manage mood and help prevent relapse?
- How can what we went over today be useful in your family?

Cognitive Restructuring and Unhelpful Thoughts

Relationship between Mood and Thoughts

- In the last session, we learned that a mood is a feeling that can be monitored.
- Our next goal is to recognize the thoughts behind our feelings.

Unhelpful Thoughts

- When depressed, your thoughts are usually negative.
- Now that you are better, some of these "leftover" negative thoughts may still be affecting your mood!

Thought Check

- **Check** the thought!
- **Challenge** the thought!
- **Change** the thought!
  - Check
    - Check to see if the thought is helpful. Check to see if the thought causes problems in mood (results in negative mood).
  - Challenge
    - Challenge the thought: Is there another way to look at this (alternatives)? What would I say to a friend who has this thought? Connect this to the triangle. How does this thought make me feel? What behavior does this thought lead to? Is this thought getting in the way of anything I want to do?
  - Change
    - Change it to be helpful.
      - Components of a good counterthought: positive, not extreme, not emotionally charged, not blaming.
- Thought Check Example: "I made a low grade on the test today, so I am going to fail the class."
  - Check
    - How did this thought make me feel?
      - Nervous about failing.
      - Worried about my parents' reaction.
      - Anxious about my future.
      - Sad because I feel stupid—everyone is smarter than I am.
  - Challenge
    - Does making a low grade automatically lead to my failing the class?
    - Have other students made low grades before and not failed?
    - Was there a reason that I did poorly?
    - **Problems have solutions!**

(continued)

- ○ Change
  - ▪ I failed a test today. However, in the future, I will get extra help and will change my study habits.

Self-Beliefs

- Self-beliefs are ideas or beliefs about oneself that contribute to negative thoughts and mood.
- Sometimes people have these recurring negative thoughts that occur daily, or even several times a day, in many situations.
  - ○ Examples include:
    - ▪ "I don't measure up."
    - ▪ "I am unlovable."
    - ▪ "I am unworthy."
  - ○ These are all examples of self-beliefs.
- One goal of this treatment is to check, challenge, and change these thoughts any time they occur.
- Doing this may be difficult, as these thoughts are most persistent.
- We will make noticing these recurring thoughts a special goal in this treatment.

Questions/Comments

- Have you noticed any negative thoughts expressed by your child lately?
- Is there a common negative thought (core belief) that your child has?
- What can the family do to help the child notice thoughts that lead to negative mood?
- How can what we went over today be useful in your family?

Problem Solving

Problems

- Everyone deals with problems and could benefit from learning how to solve them!
- "What is a problem?"
  - A problem is a source of stress.
  - Basically, a problem is any situation that causes you to be anxious, worried, or stressed out.

FLIP

- When you encounter a problem, **FLIP** the problem to look at all sides!
- **F:** Figure out what the problem is and what you want to happen.
  - Define the problem.
  - Define your goals.
- **L:** List all possible solutions.
  - Don't evaluate the solutions at this point. Just brainstorm as many as possible.
  - Remember, you have options!
- **I:** Identify the best solution.
  - Evaluate each solution.
  - Make a list of "pros" and "cons" for each solution if needed.
- **P:** Plan what to do next!
  - Define a step-by-step plan for putting your solution into place.
  - After following through with this solution, evaluate the outcome.
    - Was the outcome as you expected?
    - Did you achieve your goal?

Using FLIP

- How could FLIP have helped you in the past?
- How can this strategy help you now?

Questions/Comments

- Have you noticed any problems that FLIP could be used to solve?
- How can what we went over today be useful in your family?

Wellness

Wellness Continuum

- When people are ill, all focus shifts to the illness and less attention is paid to overall wellness and health.
- On the illness–wellness continuum, so far this treatment has focused on the illness side and on strategies targeted primarily at reducing depressive symptoms.
- It is now time to focus on the other side of this continuum—those behaviors and practices that lead to an optimal quality of life.

Wellness Skills

- Wellness skills help you "live life to the fullest!!!"
- Wellness skills are positive behaviors and attitudes that help keep you happy and healthy.

The Six S's of Wellness

- There are six general areas of wellness.
- Self-Acceptance
  - Remember to use positive self-talk to encourage yourself.
  - It is okay not to be perfect at everything.
- Social
  - Support keeps one from being stressed.
  - Friends add an aspect of fun to life!
  - Stop for a moment and consider the different friends in your life who support you in different ways.
- Success
  - Everyone likes to succeed.
  - Each person is unique and has certain strengths.
  - Remember to give yourself credit for your successes and to reward yourself!
- Self-Goals
  - Having goals gives people hope and a sense of purpose.
    - Short-term goals
    - Long-term goals
  - Consider making a list of your goals, and try to do something each week to move toward accomplishing these goals.
  - Having something to look forward to is an important aspect of keeping up hope and maintaining wellness.

(continued)

- Spiritual
  - Spiritual means different things to different people.
  - Self-awareness, including recognition of one's values and beliefs and living in conjunction with those values and beliefs, is a key part of wellness.
  - It is also important to respect the views of others (tolerance) and to participate in activities that help others (altruism) in a way to better connect to the world around you.
- Soothing
  - Stress has detrimental effects on the mind and body.
  - Relaxation is key to maintaining health.
    - What are some ways that you relax?

Development of a Wellness Plan

- Which of the six S's are you already using in your life?
- What are some areas that you need to work on?
  - Make a plan using specific examples of how you can increase the skills that you lack and how you can continue with the ones that you are already good at.

Questions/Comments

- What can the family do to help the child practice these wellness strategies?
- How can what we went over today be useful in your family?

Family Wellness

- Does your family use any of these skills?
- What are some areas that your family needs to improve?

Family Wellness Plan

- Use this space to list some wellness goals for your family.

Relapse Prevention Plan and Wellness Plan

Quick Review

- Congratulations! You have taken important steps to maintaining recovery from depression.
- Let's take a minute to review what we have covered so far in this treatment.
  - Behavioral Coping Skills
    - Some people find that doing something can immediately help with their moods.
    - We suggest:
      - Do something distracting and fun.
      - Do something relaxing and soothing.
      - Expend energy.
      - Do something social.
      - Do something that makes you feel successful: Mastery.
    - Remember to avoid things that bring your mood down (Mood Busters).
  - Thinking Differently
    - **Thought Check**
      - **Check** the thought!
      - **Challenge** the thought!
      - **Change** the thought!
    - Self-beliefs
      - Ideas or beliefs about myself that occur too often and contribute to negative thoughts and mood.
      - Remember to use Thought Check on these too!
  - Problem Solving
    - FLIP the problem to look at all sides!
      - **F:** Figure out what the problem is and what you want.
      - **L:** List all possible solutions.
      - **I:** Identify the best solution.
      - **P:** Plan what to do next.
  - Wellness Plan
    - Six general areas of wellness (the Six S's)
      - **S**elf-acceptance
      - **S**ocial
      - **S**uccess

(continued)

- □ **S**elf-goals
- □ **S**piritual
- □ **S**oothing
  - ▪ Wellness skills = positive behaviors and attitudes that help keep you happy and healthy

Relapse Prevention Plan

- Using these skills can help you to further improve and to prevent relapse.
- Do you remember the difference between a "lapse" and a "relapse"?
  - ○ Lapse versus Relapse
    - ▪ It is expected that sometimes you will have a "bad day" or be irritable or maybe even sad.
    - ▪ A **lapse** (or brief return of a depressive symptom) DOES NOT EQUAL **relapse.**
    - ▪ If there is a concern that relapse has occurred, seek treatment.
- Parts of the plan
  - ○ My signs or symptoms of a lapse.
  - ○ Skills to keep a lapse from becoming relapse.
  - ○ Personal strengths and wellness plan that keep me feeling at my best.
  - ○ The things I worry about might be difficult for me in the future (anticipated stressors).
- My child's signs/symptoms of depression
  - ○ Take a minute to list some of the symptoms that could be a **warning sign** of a lapse for your child:

_____

_____

_____

_____

_____

_____

- Skills to manage my child's signs/symptoms
  - ○ Now, look at the previous list and name some **skills** that your child could use to help manage those signs/symptoms:

_____

_____

_____

_____

_____

_____

_____

(continued)

- My child's wellness plan
  - Which of the six S's is your child already using in his or her life?

  _____

  _____

  _____

  _____

  - What are some areas that your child needs to work on, or what are his or her future wellness goals?

  _____

  _____

  _____

- Future worries
  - Can you name any concerns about things that are coming up in life that may be stressful (i.e., anticipated stressors)?

  _____

  _____

  _____

  _____

  _____

  _____

Relapse Prevention and Wellness Plan

- Ideally, this plan will help you when these future stressors occur, so that depression does not return.
- Remember, it is always okay to seek treatment if you are having trouble with your mood.
  - How can the family help prevent relapse?
- Monitor the temperature and "coaching style" of the home (see below for a reminder about this).
- Notice when good and bad things happen and listen for how your child responds.
- Praise the good! Remind your child about his or her strengths and comment when goals are achieved.
- Have a home environment that encourages wellness behaviors—for ALL members of the family!

(continued)

Family Expressed Emotion

- Family "temperature"
  - The communication and emotional level in a home can be thought of as being on a thermostat.
  - The "temperature" needs to be set at a level that is comfortable for all.
- Good coach versus bad coach
  - A good coach is supportive of the player, even when mistakes are made.
  - Good behavior is praised, and bad behavior is corrected but with support and patience.
  - "Coaching style" can be a useful metaphor for parenting style.

Questions for the Therapist

- Use this space to write down any questions you may have for today.

References

Abela, J. R. Z. (2001). The hopelessness theory of depression: A test of the diathesis–stress and causal mediation components in third and seventh grade children. *Journal of Abnormal Child Psychology, 29,* 241–254.

American Psychiatric Association. (2000). *Diagnostic and statistical manual of mental disorders* (4th ed., text rev.). Washington, DC: Author.

American Psychiatric Association. (2013). *Diagnostic and statistical manual of mental disorders* (5th ed.). Arlington, VA: Author.

Angold, A., Messer, S. C., Stangl, D., Farmer, E. M., Costello, E. J., & Burns, B. J. (1998). Perceived parental burden and service use for child and adolescent psychiatric disorders. *American Journal of Public Health, 88,* 75–80.

Asarnow, J. R., & Bates, S. (1988). Depression in child psychiatric inpatients: Cognitive and attributional patterns. *Journal of Abnormal Child Psychology, 6,* 601–615.

Asarnow, J. R., Berk, M., Hughes, J. L., & Anderson, N. L. (2015). The SAFETY Program: Ecological cognitive-behavioral intervention for adolescent suicide attempters. *Journal of Child and Adolescent Psychology, 44*(1), 194–203.

Asarnow, J. R., Goldstein, M. J., Tompson, M., & Guthrie, D. (1993). One-year outcomes of depressive disorders in child psychiatric inpatients: Evaluation of the prognostic power of a brief measure of expressed emotion. *Journal of Child Psychology and Psychiatry and Allied Disciplines, 34,* 129–137.

Asarnow, J. R., & Horton, A. A. (1990). Coping and stress in families of child psychiatric inpatients: Parents of children with depressive and schizophrenia spectrum disorders. *Child Psychiatry and Human Development, 21,* 145–157.

Asarnow, J., Jaycox, L., Clarke, G., Lewinsohn, P., Hops, H., & Rohde, P. (1999). *Stress and your mood: Teen and young adult workbook.* Unpublished manuscript.

Asarnow, J., Jaycox, L., Clarke, G., Lewinsohn, P., Hops, H., Rohde, P., et al. (2010). *Stress and your mood: A manual for individuals.* Unpublished manuscript.

Asarnow, J. R., Scott, C. V., & Mintz, J. (2002). A combined cognitive-behavioral family education intervention for depression in children: A treatment development study. *Cognitive Therapy and Research, 26,* 221–229.

Beck, A. T., Steer, R. A., & Brown, G. K. (1996). *Manual for the Beck Depression Inventory–II.* San Antonio, TX: Psychological Corporation.

Beck, A. T., Weissman, A., Lester, D., & Trexler, L. (1974). The measurement of pessimism: The Hopelessness Scale. *Journal of Consulting and Clinical Psychology, 42,* 861–865.

Beck, J. S. (1995). *Cognitive therapy: Basics and beyond.* New York: Guilford Press.

Beevers, C. G., Keitner, G. I., Ryan, C. E., & Miller, I. (2003). Cognitive predictors of symptom return following depression treatment. *Journal of Abnormal Psychology, 112,* 488–496.

Birmaher, B., Arbelaez, C., & Brent, D. (2002). Course and outcome of child and adolescent major depressive disorder. *Child and Adolescent Psychiatric Clinics of North America, 11*(3), 619–637.

Birmaher, B., Brent, D., Bernet, W., Bukstein, O., Walter, H., Benson, R. S., et al. (2007). Practice parameter for the assessment and treatment of children and adolescents with depressive disorders. *Journal of the American Academy of Child and Adolescent Psychiatry, 46*(11), 1503–1526.

Birmaher, B., Brent, D. A., Kolko, D., Baugher, M., Bridge, J., Holder, D., et al. (2000). Clinical outcome after short-term psychotherapy for adolescents with major depressive disorder. *Archives of General Psychiatry, 57,* 29–36.

Birmaher, B., Ryan, N. D., Williamson, D. E., Brent, D. A., & Kaufman, J. (1996a). Childhood and adolescent depression: A review of the past 10 years, Part II. *Journal of the American Academy of Child and Adolescent Psychiatry, 35,* 1575–1583.

Birmaher, B., Ryan, N. D., Williamson, D. E., Brent, D. A., Kaufman, J., Dahl, R. E., et al. (1996b). Childhood and adolescent depression: A review of the past 10 years, Part I. *Journal of the American Academy of Child and Adolescent Psychiatry, 35,* 1427–1439.

Birmaher, B., Williamson, D. E., Dahl, R. E., Axelson, D. A., Kaufman, J., Dorn, L. D., et al. (2004). Clinical presentation and course of depression in youth: Does onset in childhood differ from onset in adolescence? *Journal of the American Academy of Child Adolescent Psychiatry, 43*(1), 63–70.

Bockting, C., Schene, A., Spinhoven, P., Koeter, M., Wouters, L., Huyser, J., et al. (2005). Preventing relapse/recurrence in recurrent depression with cognitive therapy: A randomized controlled trial. *Journal of Consulting and Clinical Psychology, 73,* 647–657.

Brent, D., Bridge, M., & Bonner, C. (2000). *Cognitive behavior therapy manual for TORDIA.* Unpublished manuscript.

Brent, D. A., Brown, G., Curry, J. F., Goldstein, T., Hughes, J. L., Kennard, B. D., et al. (2006). *Cognitive behavior therapy for suicide prevention (CBT-SP) teen manual, version 3.* Unpublished manuscript.

Brent, D., Emslie, G., Clarke, G., Wagner, K. D., Asarnow, J. R., Keller, M., et al. (2008). Switching to another SSRI or to venlafaxine with or without cognitive behavioral therapy for adolescents with SSRI-resistant depression: The TORDIA randomized controlled trial. *Journal of the American Medical Association, 299*(8), 901–913.

Brent, D. A., Holder, D., Kolko, D., Birmaher, B., Baugher, M., Roth, C., et al. (1997). A clinical psychotherapy trial for adolescent depression comparing cognitive, family, and supportive therapy. *Archives of General Psychiatry, 54,* 877–885.

Brent, D. A., Kolko, D., Birmaher, B., Baugher, M., Bridge, J., & Roth, C. (1999). A clinical trial for adolescent depression: Predictors of additional treatment in the acute and follow-up phases of the trial. *Journal of the American Academy of Child and Adolescent Psychiatry, 38,* 263–270.

Brent, D. A., Kolko, D. J., Wartella, M. E., Boyland, M. B., Moritz, G., Baugher, M., et al. (1993). Adolescent psychiatric inpatients' risk of suicide attempt at 6-month follow-up. *Journal of the American Academy of Child and Adolescent Psychiatry, 32,* 95–105.

Brent, D. A., Perper, J. A., Goldstein, C. E., Kolko, D. J., Allan, M. J., Allman, C. J., et al. (1988). Risk factors for adolescent suicide: A comparison of adolescent suicide victims with suicidal inpatients. *Archives of General Psychiatry, 45,* 581–588.

Brent, D., & Poling, K. (1997). *Cognitive therapy treatment manual for depressed and suicidal youth.* Unpublished manuscript.

Bridge, J. A., & Brent, D. A. (2004). Adolescents with depression. *Journal of the American Medical Association, 292,* 2578.

Bridge, J. A., Goldstein, T. R., & Brent, D. A. (2006). Adolescent suicide and suicidal behavior. *Journal of Child Psychology and Psychiatry, 47*(3–4), 372–394.

Butler, L., Mietzitis, S., Friedman, R., & Cole, E. (1980). The effect of two school-based intervention programs on depressive symptoms in preadolescents. *American Educational Research Journal, 17*, 111–119.

Cheung, A. H., Emslie, G. J., & Mayes, T. L. (2005). Review of the efficacy and safety of antidepressants in youth. *Journal of Child Psychology and Psychiatry, 46*, 735–754.

Clarke, G., Debar, L., Lynch, F., Powell, J., Gale, J., O'Conner, E., et al. (2005). A randomized effectiveness trial of brief cognitive-behavioral therapy for depressed adolescents receiving antidepressant medication. *Journal of the American Academy of Child and Adolescent Psychiatry, 44*, 888–898.

Clarke, G. N., Rohde, P., Lewinsohn, P. M., Hops, H., & Seeley, J. R. (1999). Cognitive-behavioral treatment of adolescent depression: Efficacy of acute group treatment and booster sessions. *Journal of the American Academy of Child and Adolescent Psychiatry, 38*(3), 272–279.

Compton, S. N., March, J. S., Brent, D., Albano, A. M., Weersing, V. R., & Curry, J. (2004). Cognitive-behavioral psychotherapy for anxiety and depressive disorders in children and adolescents: An evidence-based medicine review. *Journal of the American Academy of Child and Adolescent Psychiatry, 43*, 930–959.

Costello, E. J., Pine, D. S., Hammen, C., March, J. S., Plotsky, P. M., Weissman, M. M., et al. (2002). Development and natural history of mood disorders. *Biological Psychiatry, 52*, 529–542.

Curry, J. F., & Craighead, W. E. (1990). Attributional style in clinically depressed and conduct disordered adolescents. *Journal of Consulting and Clinical Psychology, 58*(1), 109–115.

Curry, J., Wells, K., Brent, D., Clarke, G., Rodhe, P., Albano, A. M., et al. (2000). *Cognitive behavior therapy manual for TADS.* Unpublished manuscript.

Cusin, C., Yang, H., Yeung, A., & Fava, M. (2009). Rating scales for depression. In L. Baer & M. A. Blais (Eds.), *Handbook of clinical rating scales and assessment in psychiatry and mental health* (pp. 7–36). New York: Humana Press.

Diener, E. (1984). Subjective well-being. *Psychological Bulletin, 95*, 542–575.

Domino, M., Foster, E., Vitiello, B., Kratochvil, C., Burns, B., Silva, S., et al. (2009). Relative cost-effectiveness of treatments for adolescent depression: 36-week results from the TADS randomized trial. *Journal of the American Academy of Child and Adolescent Psychiatry, 48*(70), 711–720.

Dubicka, B., Elvins, R., Roberts, C., Chick, G., Wilkinson, P., & Goodyer, I. M. (2010). Combined treatment with cognitive-behavioural therapy in adolescent depression: meta-analysis. *British Journal of Psychiatry, 197*(6), 433–440.

Duckworth, A. L., Steen, T. A., & Seligman, M. E. (2005). Positive psychology in clinical practice. *Annual Review of Clinical Psychology, 1*(1), 629–651.

Emslie, G. J., Armitage, R., Weinberg, W. A., Rush, A. J., Mayes, T. L., & Hoffmann, R. F. (2001). Sleep polysomnography as a predictor of recurrence in children and adolescents with major depressive disorder. *International Journal of Neuropsychopharmacology, 4*(2), 159–168.

Emslie, G. J., Heiligenstein, J. H., Wagner, K. D., Hoog, S. L., Ernest, D. E., Brown, E., et al. (2002). Fluoxetine for acute treatment of depression in children and adolescents: A placebo-controlled, randomized clinical trial. *Journal of the American Academy of Child and Adolescent Psychiatry, 41*(10), 1205–1215.

Emslie, G. J., Kennard, B. D., Mayes, T. L., Nakonezny, P. A., Zhu, L., Tao, R., et al. (2012). Insomnia moderates outcome of serotonin-selective reuptake inhibitor treatment in depressed youth. *Journal of Child and Adolescent Psychopharmacology, 22*(1), 21–28.

Emslie, G. J., Kennard, B. D., Mayes, T. L., Nightingale-Teresi, J., Carmody, T., Hughes, C. W., et al. (2008). Fluoxetine versus placebo in preventing relapse of major depression in children and adolescents. *American Journal of Psychiatry, 165*(4), 459–467.

Emslie, G. J., Mayes, T. L., Laptook, R. S., & Batt, M. (2003). Predictors of response to treatment in children and adolescents with mood disorders. *Psychiatric Clinics of North America, 26*, 435–456.

Emslie, G. J., Rush, A. J., Weinberg, W. A., Gullion, C. M., Rintelmann, J., & Hughes, C. W. (1997b). Recurrence of major depressive disorder in hospitalized children and adolescents. *Journal of the American Academy of Child and Adolescent Psychiatry, 36*(6), 785–792.

Emslie, G. J., Rush, A. J., Weinberg, W. A., Kowatch, R. A., Carmody, T., & Mayes, T. L. (1998). Fluoxetine in child and adolescent depression: Acute and maintenance treatment. *Depression and Anxiety, 7,* 32–39.

Emslie, G. J., Rush, A. J., Weinberg, W. A., Kowatch, R. A., Hughes, C. W., Carmody, T., et al. (1997a). A double-blind, randomized, placebo-controlled trial of fluoxetine in children and adolescents with depression. *Archives of General Psychiatry, 54,* 1031–1037.

Fava, G. A., Fabbri, S., & Sonino, N. (2002). Residual symptoms in depression: An emerging therapeutic target. *Progress in Neuro-Psychopharmacology and Biological Psychiatry, 26,* 1019–1027.

Fava, G. A., Grandi, S., Zielezny, M., Canestrari, R., & Morphy, M. A. (1994). Cognitive behavioral treatment of residual symptoms in primary major depressive disorder. *American Journal of Psychiatry, 151,* 1295–1299.

Fava, G. A., Grandi, S., Zielezny, M., Rafanelli, C., & Canestrari, R. (1996). Four-year outcome for cognitive behavioral treatment of residual symptoms in major depression. *American Journal of Psychiatry, 153,* 945–947.

Fava, G. A., Ottolini, F., & Ruini, C. (1999). The role of cognitive behavioural therapy in the treatment of unipolar depression. *Acta Psychiatrica Scandinavica, 99*(5), 394–396.

Fava, G. A., Rafanelli, C., Grandi, S., Canestrari, R., & Morphy, M. A. (1998a). Six-year outcome for cognitive behavioral treatment of residual symptoms in major depression. *American Journal of Psychiatry, 155,* 1443–1445.

Fava, G. A., Rafanelli, C., Grandi, S., Conti, S., & Belluardo, P. (1998b). Prevention of recurrent depression with cognitive behavioral therapy: Preliminary findings. *Archives of General Psychiatry, 55*(9), 816–820.

Fava, G. A., Ruini, C., Rafanelli, C., Finos, L., Conti, S., & Grandi, S. (2004). Six-year outcome of cognitive behavior therapy for prevention of recurrent depression. *American Journal of Psychiatry, 161*(10), 1872–1876.

Fergusson, D. M., Horwood, L. J., Ridder, E.

M., & Beautrais, A. L. (2005). Subthreshold depression in adolescence and mental health outcomes in adulthood. *Archives of General Psychiatry, 62*(1), 66–72.

Food and Drug Administration. (2014). FDA: Don't leave childhood depression untreated. Retrieved from *www.fda.gov/ForConsumers/ConsumerUpdates/ucm413161.htm.*

Frank, E., Prien, R. F., Jarrett, R. B., Keller, M. B., Kupfer, D. J., Lavori, P. W., et al. (1991). Conceptualization and rationale for consensus definitions of terms in major depressive disorder. Remission, recovery, relapse, and recurrence. *Archives of General Psychiatry, 48,* 851–855.

Frisch, M. B. (2006). *Quality of life therapy.* Hoboken, NJ: Wiley.

Garber, J., Kriss, M. R., Koch, M., & Lindholm, L., (1988). Recurrent depression in adolescents: A follow-up study. *Journal of the American Academy of Child and Adolescent Psychiatry, 27,* 49–54.

Gillham, J. E., Reivich, K. J., Brunwasser, S. M., Freres, D. R., Chajon, N. D., KashMacdonald, V. M., et al. *Journal of Clinical Child and Adolescent Psychology, 41*(5), 621–639.

Gilman, R., Huebner, E. W., & Laughlin, J. E. (2000). A first study of the Multidimensional Student Life Satisfaction Scale with adolescents. *Social Indicators Research, 52,* 135–160.

Goodyer, I. M. (2002). Social adversity and mental functions in adolescents at high risk of psychopathology: Position paper and suggested framework for future research. *British Journal of Psychiatry, 181,* 383–386.

Goodyer, I. (2006). *Juvenile depression: Their nature, characteristics and outcome.* Paper presented at the 17th World Congress of the International Association for Child and Adolescent Psychiatry and Allied Professionals, Melbourne, Australia.

Gotlib, I. H., Lewinsohn, P. M., Seeley, J. R., Rohde, P., & Redner, J. E. (1993). Negative cognitions and attributional style in depressed adolescents: An examination of stability and specificity. *Journal of Abnormal Psychology, 102,* 607–615.

Guidi, J., Fava, G. A., Fava, M., & Papakostas, G. I. (2011). Efficacy of the sequential integration of psychotherapy and pharmacotherapy in major depressive disorder: A preliminary meta-analysis. *Psychological Medicine, 41*(2), 321–331.

Haby, M. M., Tonge, B., Littlefield, L., Carter, R., & Vos, T. (2004). Cost-effectivness of cognitive behavioral therapy and selective serotonin reuptake inhibitors of major depression in children and adolescents. *Australian and New Zealand Journal of Psychiatry, 38,* 579–591.

Hammen, C. (1992). Life events and depression: The plot thickens. *American Journal of Community Psychology, 20,* 179–193.

Harrington, R., Fudge, H., Rutter, M., Pickles, A., & Hill, J. (1990). Adult outcomes of childhood and adolescent depression: I. Psychiatric status. *Archives of General Psychiatry, 47,* 465–473.

Hollon, S. D., DeRubeis, R. J., Shelton, R. C., Amsterdam, J. D., Salomon, R. M., O'Reardon, J. P., et al. (2005). Prevention of relapse following cognitive therapy vs. medications in moderate to severe depression. *Archives of General Psychiatry, 62,* 417–422.

Huebner, E. S. (1994). Preliminary development and validation of a multidimensional life satisfaction scale for children. *Psychological Assessment, 6,* 149–158.

Jarrett, R. B. (2001). *Continuation therapy for major depressive disorder.* Unpublished manuscript.

Jarrett, R. B., & Kraft, D. (1997). Prophylactic cognitive therapy for major depressive disorder. *In Session, 3,* 55–67.

Jarrett, R. B., Kraft, D., Doyle, J., Foster, B. M., Eaves, G. G., & Silver, P. C. (2001). Preventing recurrent depression using cognitive therapy with and without a continuation phase:A randomized clinical trial. *Archives of General Psychiatry, 58*(4), 381–388.

Jarrett, R. B., Minhajuddin, A., Gershenfeld, H., Friedman, E. S., & Thase, M. E. (2013). Preventing depressive relapse and recurrence in higher-risk cognitive therapy responders: A randomized trial of continuation phase cognitive therapy, fluoxetine, or matched pill placebo. *Journal of the American Medical Association, 70*(11), 1152–1160.

Jaycox, L. H., Reivich, K. J., Gillham, J., & Seligman, M. E. (1994). Prevention of depressive symptoms in school children. *Behaviour Research and Therapy, 32,* 801–816.

Johnson, J. G., Spitzer, R. S., Kroenke, K., & Williams, J. B. W. (2005). *The Patient Health Questionnaire for Adolescents, Revised Version (PHQ-A).* New York: Biometrics Research Department, New York State Psychiatric Institute.

Kahn, J. S., Kehle, T. J., Jenson, W. R., & Clark, E. (1990). Comparison of cognitive-behavioral, relaxation, and self-modeling interventions for depression among middle-school students. *School Psychology Review, 19,* 196–211.

Kandel, D. B., & Davies, M. (1986). Adult sequelae of adolescent depressive symptoms. *Archives of General Psychiatry, 43,* 255–262.

Karp, J., Buysse, D., Houck, P., Cherry, C., Kupfer, D., & Frank, E. (2004). Relationship of variability in residual symptoms with recurrence of major depressive disorder during maintenance treatment. *American Journal of Psychiatry, 161,* 1877–1884.

Kaslow, N. J., Stark, K. D., Printz, B., Livingston, R., & Tsai, S. (1992). Cognitive Triad Inventory for Children: Development and relationship to depression and anxiety. *Journal of Clinical Child Psychology, 21,* 339–347.

Kaufman, J., Birmaher, B., Brent, D., Rao, U., Flynn, C., Moreci, P., et al. (1997). Schedule for Affective Disorders and Schizophrenia for School-Age Children–Present and Lifetime version (K-SADS-PL): Initial reliability and validity data. *Journal of the American Academy of Child and Adolescent Psychiatry, 36,* 980–988.

Kaufman, J., Martin, A., King, R. A., & Charney, D. (2001). Are child-, adolescent-, and adult-onset depression one and the same disorder? *Biological Psychiatry, 49*(12), 980–1001.

Kaufman, J., Yang, B., Douglas-Palumberi, H., Houshyar, S., Lipschitz, D., Krystal, J. H., et al. (2004). Social supports and serotonin transporter gene moderate depression in maltreated children. *Proceedings of the National Academy of Sciences, 101,* 17316–17321.

Kazdin, A. E., French, N. H., Unis, A. S., Esveldt-Dawson, K., & Sherick, R. B. (1983). Hopelessness, depression, and suicidal intent among psychiatrically disturbed inpatient children. *Journal of Consulting and Clinical Psychology, 51,* 504–510.

Keller, M. B., Ryan, N., Strober, M., Klein, R. G., Kutcher, S., Birmaher, B., et al. (2001). Efficacy of paroxetine in the treatment of adolescent major depression: A randomized, controlled trial. *Journal of the American Academy of Child and Adolescent Psychiatry, 40,* 762–772.

Kennard, B. D., Emslie, G. J., Mayes, T. L., Nakonezny, P. A., Jones, J. M., Foxwell, A. A., et al. (2014). Sequential treatment with fluoxetine and relapse—prevention CBT to improve outcomes in pediatric depression. *American Journal of Psychiatry, 171*(10), 1083–1090.

Kennard, B. D., Emslie, G. J., Mayes, T. L., Nightingale-Teresi, J., Nakonezny, P. A., Hughes, J. L., et al. (2008a). Cognitive-behavioral therapy to prevent relapse in pediatric responders to pharmacotherapy for major depressive disorder. *Journal of the American Academy of Child and Adolescent Psychiatry, 47*(12), 1395–1404.

Kennard, B. D., & Rush, A. J. (1995). *Managing your depression: A guide for teenagers* [pamphlet]. Dallas: University of Texas Southwestern Medical Center.

Kennard, B., Silva, S., Vitiello, B., Curry, J., Kratochvil, C., Simons, A., et al. (2006). Remission and residual symptoms after acute treatment of adolescents with major depressive disorder. *Journal of the American Academy of Child and Adolescent Psychiatry, 45,* 1404–1411.

Kennard, B. D., Stewart, S. M., Hughes, J. L., Jarrett, R. B., & Emslie, G. J. (2008b). Developing cognitive behavioral therapy to prevent depressive relapse in youth. *Cognitive and Behavioral Practice, 15,* 387–399.

Klein, D. N., Dougherty, L. R., & Olino, T. M. (2005). Toward guidelines for evidence-based assessment of depression in children and adolescents. *Journal of Clinical Child and Adolescent Psychology, 34*(3), 412–432.

Klein, D. N., Lewinsohn, P. M., Seeley, J. R., & Rohde, P. (2001). A family study of major depressive disorder in a community sample of adolescents. *Archives of General Psychiatry, 58,* 13–20.

Klein, J. B., Jacobs, R. H., & Reinecke, M. A. (2007). Cognitive-behavioral therapy for adolescent depression: A meta-analytic investigation of changes in effect-size estimates. *Journal of the American Academy of Child and Adolescent Psychiatry, 46*(11), 1403–1413.

Kobau, R., Seligman, M. E., Peterson, C., Diener, E., Zack, M. M., Chapman, D., et al. (2011). Mental health promotion in public health: Perspectives and strategies from positive psychology. *American Journal of Public Health, 101*(8), e1–e9.

Koeppen, A. S. (1974). Relaxation training for children. *Elementary School Guidance and Counseling, 9,* 14–21.

Kovacs, M. (1992). *Children's Depression Inventory (CDI) manual.* Toronto: Multi-Health Systems.

Kovacs, M. (2010). *The Children's Depression Inventory, Second Edition (CDI-2).* North Tonawanda, NY: Multi-Health Systems.

Kovacs, M., Akiskal, H. S., Gatsonis, C., & Parrone, P. L. (1994). Childhood-onset dysthymic disorder: Clinical features and prospective naturalistic outcome. *Archives of General Psychiatry, 51,* 365–374.

Kovacs, M., Feinberg, T. L., Crouse-Novak, M. A., Paulauskas, S. L., & Finkelstein, R. (1984a). Depressive disorders in childhood: I. A longitudinal prospective study of characteristics and recovery. *Archives of General Psychiatry, 41,* 229–237.

Kovacs, M., Feinberg, T. L., Crouse-Novak, M. A., Paulauskas, S. L., Pollock, M., & Finkelstein, R. (1984b). Depressive disorders in childhood: II. A longitudinal study of the risk for a subsequent major depression. *Archives of General Psychiatry, 41,* 643–649.

Kroenke, K., Spitzer, R. L., & Williams, J. B. (2001). The PHQ-9: Validity of a brief depression severity measure. *Journal of General Internal Medicine, 16*(9), 606–613.

Kroll, L., Harrington, R., Jayson, D., Fraser, J., & Gowers, S. (1996). Pilot study of continuation cognitive-behavioral therapy for major depression in adolescent psychiatric patients. *Journal of the American Academy of Child and Adolescent Psychiatry, 35,* 1156–1161.

Kumar, G., Steer, R. A., Teitelman, K. B., & Villacis, L. (2002). Effectiveness of Beck Depression Inventory–II subscales in screening for major depressive disorders in adolescent psychiatric inpatients. *Assessment, 9*(2), 164–170.

Kupfer, D. J. (1991). Long-term treatment of depression. *Journal of Clinical Psychiatry, 52* (Suppl. 5), 28–34.

Lerner, M. S., & Clum, G. A. (1990). Treatment of suicide ideators: A problem-solving approach. *Behavior Therapy, 21,* 403–411.

Lewinsohn, P. M., Allen, N. B., Seeley, J. R., & Gotlib, I. H. (1999). First onset versus recurrence of depression: Differential processes of psychosocial risk. *Journal of Abnormal Psychology, 108*, 483–489.

Lewinsohn, P. M., Clarke, G. N., Hops, H., & Andrews, J. A. (1990). Cognitive-behavioral treatment for depressed adolescents. *Behavior Therapy, 21*, 385–401.

Lewinsohn, P. M., Hops, H., Roberts, R. E., Seeley, J. R., & Andrews, J. A., (1993). Adolescent psychopathology: I. Prevalence and incidence of depression and other DSM-III-R disorders in high school students. *Journal of Abnormal Psychology, 102*(1), 135–144.

Lewinsohn, P. M., Pettit, J. W., Joiner, T. E., Jr., & Seeley, J. R. (2003). The symptomatic expression of major depressive disorder in adolescents and young adults. *Journal of Abnormal Psychology, 112*(2), 244–252.

Liddle, B., & Spence, S. H. (1990). Cognitive-behaviour therapy with depressed primary school children: A cautionary note. *Behavioural Psychotherapy, 18*, 85–102.

Luby, J. L., Mrakotsky, C., Heffelfinger, A., Brown, K., & Spitznagel, E. (2004). Characteristics of depressed preschoolers with and without anhedonia: Evidence for a melancholic depressive subtype in young children. *American Journal of Psychiatry, 161*(11), 1998–2004.

March, J., Silva, S., Petrycki, S., Curry, J., Wells, K., Fairbank, J., et al. (2004). Fluoxetine, cognitive-behavioral therapy, and their combination for adolescents with depression: Treatment for Adolescents with Depression Study (TADS) randomized controlled trial. *Journal of the American Medical Association, 292*(7), 807–820.

McCauley, E., Mitchell, J. R., Burke, P. M., & Moss, S. J. (1988). Cognitive attributes of depression in children and adolescents. *Journal of Consulting and Clinical Psychology, 56*, 903–908.

McCauley, E., Myers, K., Mitchell, J., Calderon, R., Schloredt, K., & Treder, R. (1993). Depression in young people: Initial presentation and clinical course. *Journal of the American Academy of Child and Adolescent Psychiatry, 32*, 714–722.

McCullough, M. E. (1999). Research on religion-accommodative counseling: Review and meta-analysis. *Journal of Counseling Psychology, 46*, 92–98.

Montgomery, S., Doogan, D., & Burnside, R.

(1991). The influence of different relapse criteria on the assessment of long-term efficacy of sertraline. *International Clinical Psychopharmacology, 6*(Suppl. 2), 37–46.

Morin, A. J., Moullec, G., Maiano, C., Layet, L., & Ninot, G. (2011). Psychometric properties of the Center for Epidemiologic Studies Depression Scale (CES-D) in French clinical and nonclinical adults. *Revue d'Épidémiologie et de Santé Publique, 59*(5), 327–340.

Naicker, K., Galambos, N. L., Zeng, Y., Senthilselvan, A., & Colman, I. (2013). Social, demographic, and health outcomes in the 10 years following adolescent depression. *Journal of Adolescent Health, 52*(5), 533–538.

National Mental Health Association. (2004). Depression and children. Retrieved September 8, 2004, from *www.nmha.org/children/children_mh_matters/depression.cfm*.

Nemeroff, C. B., Heim, C. M., Thase, M. E., Klein, D. N., Rush, A. J., Schatzberg, A. F., et al. (2003). Differential responses to psychotherapy versus pharmacotherapy in patients with chronic forms of major depression and childhood trauma. *Proceedings of the National Academy of Sciences, 100*, 14293–14296.

Nierenberg, A. A. (2001). Long-term management of chronic depression. *Journal of Clinical Psychiatry, 62*, 17–21.

Pargament, K. I., & Mahoney, A. (2005). Sacred matters: Sanctification as a vital topic for the psychology of religion. *International Journal for the Psychology of Religion, 15*, 179–198.

Paykel, E. S. (2007). Cognitive therapy in relapse prevention in depression. *International Journal of Neuropsychopharmacology, 10*(1), 131–136.

Paykel, E. S., Scott, J., Teasdale, J. D., Johnson, A. L., Garland, A., Moore, R., et al. (1999). Prevention of relapse in residual depression by cognitive therapy: A controlled trial. *Archives of General Psychiatry, 56*, 829–835.

Pence, B. W., Gaynes, B. N., Williams, Q., Modi, R., Adams, J., Quinlivan, E. B., et al. (2012). Assessing the effect of measurement-based care depression treatment on HIV medication adherence and health outcomes: Rationale and design of the SLAM DUNC Study. *Contemporary Clinical Trials, 33*(4), 828–838.

Perlis, R., Nierenberg, A., Alpert, J., Pava, J.,

Matthews, J., Buchin, J., et al. (2002). The effects of adding cognitive therapy to fluoxetine dose increase on risk of relapse and residual depressive symptoms in continuation treatment of major depressive disorder. *Journal of Clinical Psychopharmacology, 22,* 474–480.

Perou, R., Bitsko, R. H., Blumberg, S. J., Pastor, P., Ghandour, R. M., Gfroerer, J. C., et al. (2013). Mental health surveillance among children: United States, 2005–2011. *MMWR Surveillance Summary, 62*(Suppl. 2), 1–35.

Petersen, T., Harley, R., Papakostas, G. I., Montoya, H. D., Fava, M., & Alpert, J. E. (2004). Continuation cognitive-behavioural therapy maintains attributional style improvement in depressed patients responding acutely to fluoxetine. *Psychological Medicine, 34*(3), 555–561.

Poling, K., & Brent, D. (1997). *Living with depression: A survival manual for families.* Pittsburgh: University of Pittsburgh Health System Services for Teens at Risk.

Posner, K., Brent, D., Lucas, C., Gould, M., Stanley B., Brown, G., et al. (2008). *Columbia–Suicide Severity Rating Scale (C-SSRS).* New York: Research Foundation for Mental Hygiene.

Posner, K., Brown, G. K., Stanley, B., Brent, D. A., Yershova, K. V., Oquendo, M. A., et al. (2011). The Columbia–Suicide Severity Rating Scale: Initial validity and internal consistency findings from three multisite studies with adolescents and adults. *American Journal of Psychiatry, 168*(12), 1266–1277.

Propst, L. R., Ostrom, R., Watkins, P., Dean, T., & Mashburn, D. (1992). Comparative efficacy of religious and nonreligious cognitive-behavioral therapy for the treatment of clinical depression in religious individuals. *Journal of Consulting and Clinical Psychology, 60,* 94–103.

Radloff, L. S. (1977). The CES-D scale: A self report depression scale for research in the general population. *Applied Psychological Measurement, 1,* 385–401.

Rao, U., Hammen, C., & Daley, S. (1999). Continuity of depression during the transition to adulthood: A 5-year longitudinal study of young women. *Journal of the American Academy of Child and Adolescent Psychiatry, 38*(7), 908–915.

Rao, U., Neal, R. D., Birmaher, B., Dahl, R. E.,

Williamson, D. E., Kaufman, J., et al. (1995). Unipolar depression in adolescents: Clinical outcome in adulthood. *Journal of the American Academy of Child and Adolescent Psychiatry, 34,* 566–578.

Reynolds, W. M., & Coats, K. I. (1986). A comparison of cognitive-behavioral therapy and relaxation training for the treatment of depression in adolescents. *Journal of Consulting and Clinical Psychology, 54,* 653–660.

Rohde, P., Lewinsohn, P. M., & Seeley, J. R. (1994). Are adolescents changed by an episode of major depression? *Journal of the American Academy of Child and Adolescent Psychiatry, 33,* 1289–1298.

Rosello, J., & Bernal, G. (1999). The efficacy of cognitive-behavioral and interpersonal treatments for depression in Puerto Rican adolescents. *Journal of Consulting and Clinical Psychology, 67,* 734–745.

Rush, A. J., Crismon, M. L., Toprac, M. G., Trivedi, M. H., Rago, W. V., Shon, S., et al. (1998). Consensus guidelines in the treatment of major depressive disorder. *Journal of Clinical Psychiatry, 59*(Suppl. 20), 73–84.

Rush, A. J., Kraemer, H. C., Sackeim, H. S., Fava, M., Trivedi, M. H., Frank, E., et al. (2006). Report by the ACNP Task Force on response and remission in major depressive disorder. *Neuropsychopharmacology, 31,* 1841–1853.

Rush, A. J., Trivedi, M. H., Ibrahim, H. M., Carmody, T. J., Arnow, B., Klein, D. N., et al. (2003). The 16-item Quick Inventory of Depressive Symptomatology (QIDS), clinician rating (QIDS-C), and self-report (QIDS-SR): A psychometric evaluation in patients with chronic major depression. *Biological Psychiatry, 54,* 573–583.

Ryff, C. D., & Singer, B. (1996). Psychological well-being: Meaning, measurement, and implications for psychotherapy research. *Psychotherapy and Psychosomatics, 65,* 14–23.

Scott, J., Palmer, S., Paykel, E., Teasdale, J., & Hayhurst, H. (2003). Use of cognitive therapy for relapse prevention in chronic depression: Cost-effectiveness study. *British Journal of Psychiatry, 182,* 221–227.

Segal, Z. V., Williams, J. M. G., & Teasdale, J. D. (2002). *Mindfulness-based cognitive therapy for Depression: A new approach to preventing relapse.* New York: Guilford Press.

Seligman, M. E., & Csikszentmihalyi, M.

(2000). Positive psychology: An introduction. *American Psychologist, 55*(1), 5–14.

Seligman, M. E. P., Schulman, P., DeRubeis, R. J., & Hollon, S. D. (1999). The prevention of depression and anxiety. *Prevention and Treatment, 2* (1), Article 8a. Available at *http://journals.apa.org/prevention/volume2/pre0020008a.html*.

Seligman, M. E. P., Steen, T. A., Park, N., & Peterson, C. (2005). Positive psychology progress: Empirical validation of interventions. *American Psychologist, 60*(5), 410–421.

Shaffer, D., Gould, M. S., Brasic, J., Ambrosini, P., Fisher, P., Bird, H., et al. (1983). A children's global assessment scale (CGAS). *Archives of General Psychiatry, 40*(11), 1228–1231.

Shaffer, D., Gould, M. S., Fisher, P., Tautman, P., Moreau, D., Kleinman, M., et al. (1996). Psychiatric diagnosis in child and adolescent suicide. *Archives of General Psychiatry, 53*, 339–348.

Sin, N. L., & Lyubomirsky, S. (2009). Enhancing well-being and alleviating depressive symptoms with positive psychology interventions: A practice-friendly meta-analysis. *Journal of Clinical Psychology, 65*(5), 467–487.

Snyder, C. R., & Lopez, S. J. (Eds.). (2005). *Handbook of positive psychology.* New York: Oxford University Press.

Stark, K. D., Reynolds, W. M., & Kaslow, N. J. (1987). A comparison of the relative efficacy of self-control therapy and a behavioral problem-solving therapy for depression in children. *Journal of Abnormal Child Psychology, 15*, 91–113.

Stark, K. D., Schnoebelen, S., Simpson, J., Hargrave, J., & Glen, R. (2007a). *Treating depressed children: Therapist manual for "ACTION."* Ardmore, PA: Workbook Publishing.

Stark, K. D., Schnoebelen, S., Simpson, J., Hargrave, J., Molnar, J. & Glen, R. (2007b). *Treating depressed youth: Therapist manual for "ACTION."* Ardmore, PA: Workbook Publishing.

Stark, K. D., Simpson, J., Schnoebelen, S., Glen, R., & Hargrave, J. (2007c). *ACTION workbook.* Ardmore, PA: Workbook Publishing.

Strober, M., Lampert, C., Schmidt-Lackner, S., & Morrell, W. (1993). The course of major depressive disorder in adolescents: I. Recovery and risk of manic switching in a follow-up of

psychotic and nonpsychotic subtypes. *Journal of the American Academy of Child and Adolescent Psychiatry, 32*(1), 34–42.

Sturm, R., & Wells, K. B. (1995). How can care for depression become more cost-effective? *Journal of the American Medical Association, 273*, 51–58.

TADS Team. (2004). Fluoxetine, cognitive-behavioral therapy, and their combination for adolescents with depression: Treatment for Adolescents with Depression Study (TADS) randomized controlled trial. *Journal of the American Medical Association, 292*, 807–820.

Tao, R., Mayes, T., Hughes, C., Rintelmann, J., & Emslie, G. (2005, October). *Remission rates of depressed youth over 12-week acute fluoxetine treatment.* Abstracted in the Scientific Proceedings of the 52nd Annual Meeting, American Academy of Child and Adolescent Psychiatry, Toronto.

Teasdale, J. D., Scott, J., Moore, R. G., Hayhurst, H., Pope, M., & Paykel, E. S. (2001). How does cognitive therapy prevent relapse in residual depression? Evidence from a controlled trial. *Journal of Consulting and Clinical Psychology, 69*, 347–357.

Teasdale, J. D., Segal, Z. V., Williams, J. M., Ridgeway, V. A., Soulsby, J. M., & Lau, M. A. (2000). Prevention of relapse/recurrence in major depression by mindfulness-based cognitive therapy. *Journal of Consulting and Clinical Psychology, 68*, 615–623.

Tems, C. L., Stewart, S. M., Skinner, J. R., Hughes, C. W., & Emslie, G. J. (1993). Cognitive distortions in depressed children and adolescents: Are they state dependent or trait-like? *Journal of Clinical Child Psychology, 22*, 316–326.

Trivedi, M. H. (2009). Tools and strategies for ongoing assessment of depression: A measurement-based approach to remission. *Journal of Clinical Psychiatry, 70*(Suppl. 6), 26–31.

Vitiello, B., Rohde, P., Silva, S. G., Wells, K. C., Casat, C., Waslick, B. D., et al. (2006). Functioning and quality of life in the Treatment for Adolescents with Depression Study (TADS). *Journal of the American Academy of Child and Adolescent Psychiatry, 45*, 1419–1426.

Vostanis, P., Feehan, C., Grattan, E. F., & Bickerton, W. L. (1996). A randomised controlled outpatient trial of cognitive-behavioural treatment for children and adolescents with depression: 9-month follow-up. *Journal of Affective Disorders, 40*, 105–116.

Wagner, K. D., Ambrosini, P. J., Rynn, M., Wohlberg, C., Ruoyong, Y., Greenbaum, M. S., et al. (2003). Efficacy of sertraline in the treatment of children and adolescents with major depressive disorder. *Journal of the American Medical Association, 290*(8), 1033–1041.

Wagner, K. D., Robb, A. S., Findling, R. L., Jin, J., Gutierrez, M. M., & Heydom, W. E. (2004). A randomized, placebo-controlled trial of citalopram for the treatment of major depression in children and adolescents. *American Journal of Psychiatry, 161*, 1079–1083.

Weissman, M. M., Wolk, S., Goldstein, R. B., Moreau, D., Adams, P., Greenwald, S., et al. (1999b). Depressed adolescents grownup. *Journal of the American Medical Association, 281*, 1707–1713.

Weissman, M. M., Wolk, S., Wickramaratne, P., Goldstein, R., Adams, P., Greenwald, S., et al. (1999a). Children with prepubertal-onset major depressive disorder and anxiety grown up. *Archives of General Psychiatry, 56*, 794–801.

Weisz, J. R., McCarty, C. A., & Valeri, S. M. (2006). Effects of psychotherapy for depression in children and adolescents: A meta-analysis. *Psychological Bulletin, 132*, 132–149.

Weisz, J. R., Thurber, C. A., Sweeney, L., Proffitt, V. D., & LeGagnoux, G. L. (1997). Brief treatment of mild-to-moderate child depression using primary and secondary control enhancement training. *Journal of Consulting and Clinical Psychology, 65*, 703–707.

Wilkes, T. C. R., Belsher, G., Rush, A. J., & Frank, E. (1994). *Cognitive therapy for depressed adolescents.* New York: Guilford Press.

Wood, A., Harrington, R., & Moore, A. (1996). Controlled trial of a brief cognitive-behavioural intervention in adolescent patients with depressive disorders. *Journal of Child Psychology and Psychiatry and Allied Disciplines, 37*, 737–746.

Yorbik, O., Birmaher, B., Axelson, D., Williamson, D. E., & Ryan, N. D. (2004). Clinical characteristics of depressive symptoms in children and adolescents with major depressive disorder. *Journal of Clinical Psychiatry, 65*(12), 1654–1659; quiz 1760–1761.

Index

Note. *f* or *t* following a page number indicates a figure or a table.